The Secret of Permanent Weight Loss

PREVIEW

YOUR PERSONAL GUIDE ON HOW TO LOSE WEIGHT EFFECTIVELY AND KEEP IT OFF PERMANENTLY

THIS BOOK INVESTIGATES AND ANSWERS THE FOLLOWING QUESTIONS:

- *What are the most common causes of obesity?*

- *Why do conventional diets fail in the long run?*

- *Do we need to exercise at all?*

- *How to lose weight permanently without dieting?*

- *What is the secret of human longevity and health?*

- *How was real science hijacked by junk science, and why were we given bad diet advice for decades?*

THE SECRET OF

PERMANENT
WEIGHT LOSS

WHAT YOUR DOCTOR
WON'T TELL YOU

DR. THOMAS TOROK

CONTENTS

INTRODUCTION

Obesity is the plague of the new millennium. Since the beginning of the 20th century, obesity has claimed more lives than all wars, violent events and dictatorships combined, including World War I, World War II, genocides, civil wars, man-made famines and communism. The vast majority of our modern-day diseases such as type-2 diabetes, heart disease, stroke, cancer, arthritis and many others are closely related to obesity. The common feature of these ailments is that they are all lifestyle diseases and in many cases they could be prevented by simply adopting a healthy lifestyle.

Have you ever wondered, why are there fat doctors? Physicians treat all sorts of diseases; they are the experts of the physiology of the human body. However, despite their expertise, they are just as obese as the rest of us. Have you ever wondered if we were given the wrong advice? How does mainstream medicine treat obesity? What kind of guidance were we given? Eat less, exercise more. Avoid fat, eat more fruits and vegetables. Count calories. Drink four glasses of milk every day. Eat six meals a day. Snack between meals. Take multivitamins, mineral supplements. It's the perfect recipe for disaster, as people are just getting more and more obese every year. Obviously, we have lost the battle against obesity. But why did that happen? It seems like real science got hijacked by junk science, and we were given bad diet advice for decades.

Mainstream medicine heavily relies on a very controversial theory, called the *diet-heart hypothesis*. The whole idea is based on two key assumptions: One; dietary fat raises blood cholesterol levels; Two; high blood cholesterol increases the risk of heart disease. Cholesterol earned a very bad reputation during the past couple of decades. It should be noted that cholesterol is often confused with the *low density lipoprotein* known as LDL, which is also referred to as the "bad cholesterol". Although there is some moderate correlation between LDL levels and cardiovascular disease, the relationship is much weaker than previously thought. Cholesterol by itself is absolutely harmless, it plays many important functions and is present in every single cell of our body. Literally, there is no life without cholesterol. It is never mentioned in mainstream media, that dietary fat and cholesterol intake has virtually zero effect on your blood cholesterol level. Since its conception, the *diet-heart hypothesis* has lacked scientific evidence. In the beginning of the great coronary heart disease epidemic of the 1960s however, the *diet-heart hypothesis* had become more like a political issue. The long debate about the harmful effect of *refined carbohydrates* vs. *fats* was finally decided by politicians, not by scientists.

In 1977, the Nutrition Committee of the *United States Senate* published a pamphlet entitled *Dietary Goals for the United States*. This was the first time in history that the government told people to reduce their fat consumption and increase their carbohydrate intake. Unfortunately, people took the bad advice and did exactly what they were told to do. The fattening effect of carbohydrates was suddenly forgotten. Dietary fat and cholesterol became the number one public enemy. During the dark ages of fat phobia, renowned biochemist, *David Kritchevsky*, once controversially stated: "In America, we no longer fear God or the communists, but we fear fat". As we followed the wrong advice and went low fat, we increased our carbohydrate consumption and also developed the new habit of constant "grazing", we just became more and more obese. Since the 1970s, the number of obese individuals has tripled. Overweight people, including the obese make up 70% of the U.S. population today.

This is not just a regular diet book, but a comprehensive study on the causes and treatment of obesity. Personally, I do not believe in dieting at all. Diets simply fail in the long run, all of them. Once the program is over, within a few months or a year, the pounds gradually will come back. In order to achieve long-lasting results, you need to completely change your lifestyle; a temporary fix is not enough. In this book, I will share with you the secret of permanent weight loss. Obesity, diabetes, cardiovascular disease and many modern-day ailments have the same underlying cause: an unhealthy lifestyle. If you treat the roots of these conditions, you will not only get rid of your extra pounds, but you will also prevent most of our modern-day lifestyle diseases.

INTRODUCTION

This book summarizes four years of my research. I have a Ph.D. degree in Nutrition Science. All my statements are backed with scientific evidence, see the *Endnotes* section. The weight-loss plans described in this book are not only scientifically proven, but I also tested them personally. I was the very first subject myself. In *Chapter 52* you can read my story, how I managed to lose and keep off 55 pounds in total.

Just like in a good movie, the best part comes at the end. If you are eager to decode the secret of permanent weight loss, you can jump right to *chapter 41,* entitled *The Five Pillars of Health* and read until the end of the book. Under no circumstances, should you miss *chapters 22 to 39.* They will guide you through the jungle that is the food industry and help you make wise choices on what foods are good for you and what you should avoid. The discussions and scientific explanations can be found in *chapters 7-15.* All of my research is summarized in *chapter 15,* which explains the actual cause of today's obesity epidemic. Please don't miss this one. The rest of the book contains lots of useful information on the scientific, economic and political aspects of obesity.

I wish you best of luck on your weight-loss journey and becoming a healthier person.

With regards,

Thomas Torok, Ph.D.
Barrie, Ontario, Canada, 2020

PART

ONE

THE OBESITY EPIDEMIC

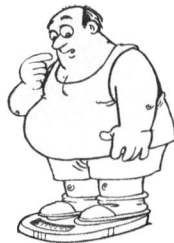

1

THE PLAGUE OF THE 21ˢᵀ CENTURY

THE EPIDEMIC

The *World Health Organization* (WHO) calls obesity a *worldwide epidemic*. The number of obese people around the world has increased dramatically over the last four decades. Since 1975, the rate of worldwide obesity has nearly tripled. In 2016, over 1.9 billion adults were overweight. More than 650 million of these adults were obese.[1] Obesity is increasing at an alarming rate among children and adolescents; 340 million of them were overweight or obese in 2016.

Over the course of the past four decades the *body mass index* of both men and women has been steadily increasing in virtually every single industrialized country (see Figure 1.1). France and Switzerland are the only places where the average BMI of women is pretty much the same as it was 40 years ago. More surprisingly, there is a third country, where BMIs are actually even lower than in the 1970s. Japanese women tend to be thinner even than 40 years ago. As for the rest of the world, we are just getting bigger and bigger.

Theatre Projects is a well-known international company specializing in the planning and building of theatres, opera houses, concert halls and corporate auditoriums. They have designed over 1,500 performing arts facilities worldwide. In 2010, an article was published in the *Wall Street Journal* entitled "Playing to Plumper Audiences" on the necessary upsizing of theatre seats in the United States.[2] Theatre experts say that due to the current rise in obesity over the last decades, the standard width of the seats had to be revised. While in the 19ᵗʰ century, theatre seats were typically 19 inches wide, by the end of the last century the width of the seats grew to 21 inches. Recently the width of regular theatre seats has been standardized at 22 inches. In addition to the wider seats, the spacing between the rows has

Body Mass Index, Men

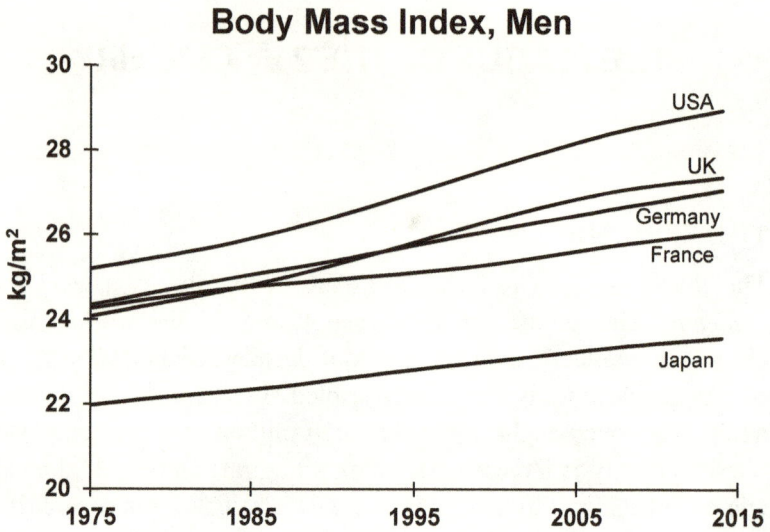

Body Mass Index, Women

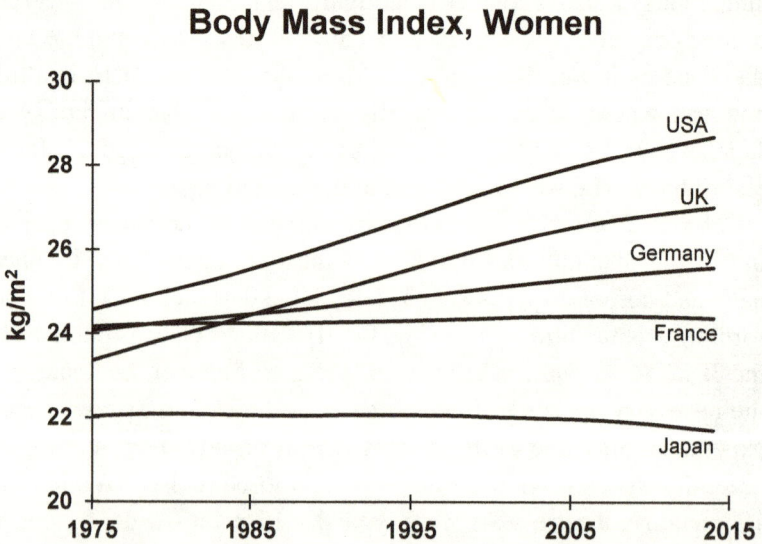

Figure 1.1. Change in body mass index between 1975-2014

largely increased as well. Since the early 20th century, theatergoers have gotten a lot bigger. Similar auditoriums built a century ago could hold twice the number of patrons as compared to the ones designed today.

The United States has the highest obesity rate among any industrialized country. In 2016, 36% of Americans were obese. Since the 1970s, the number of obese people has tripled. Overweight individuals, including the obese make up 70% of the U.S. population.[3]

THE DEADLY QUARTET

The importance of maintaining a healthy weight goes far beyond aesthetics. Obesity is associated with a wide range of diseases and health conditions. *Obesity, high blood pressure, diabetes* and *high blood triglyceride levels* are considered by scientists the major risk factors for coronary heart disease, and are often referred to as *"The Deadly Quartet"*. Hypertension with associated cardiovascular disorders is the main consequence of obesity. Clinical studies have proven that maintaining a low body mass index, preferably below 25, is the most effective primary prevention measure of hypertension.

Type-2 diabetes and obesity go hand in hand; usually people with type-2 diabetes are also obese. Researchers studied the risk of developing type-2 diabetes among thin and obese men and women. Severely obese women (BMI>35) are *93 times more likely* to develop diabetes than lean women (BMI<22). As for men, the risk ratio of becoming diabetic is *42 times higher* for the severely obese than for the normal weight.[4] Type-2 diabetes and heart disease are the most devastating disorders associated with obesity. In addition to that, certain cancers, such as stomach, colon, rectum, pancreas, gallbladder, liver, kidney, uterus, ovary and prostate cancer are closely related to obesity: they account for one fifth of all cancer deaths.

It is a well-known fact that heavy alcohol use leads to a buildup of fat inside the liver cells, a condition called *fatty liver disease*. What is less well-known however, is that even those who don't drink alcohol at all can also develop fatty liver disease. The liver is the largest organ of the human body. It plays an important role in digestion,

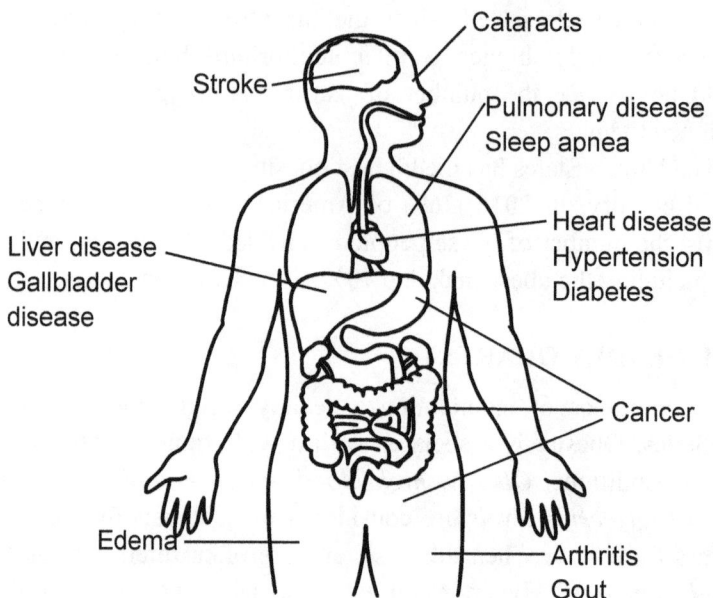

Figure 1.2. Diseases associated with obesity

energy storage and the removal of toxic substances. Both *alcohol-related fatty liver disease* and *nonalcoholic fatty liver disease* are serious conditions. In the case of alcoholic fatty liver disease, damage is caused by alcohol-induced toxicity; in the case of nonalcoholic fatty liver disease, damage is caused by lipotoxicity that results from excessive fat accumulation in the body.

Stroke is the third most common cause of death worldwide after coronary artery disease and cancer. Obesity significantly increases the risk of stroke due to a constant state of low-grade inflammation caused by excess body fat. In addition to the continuous inflammation caused by obesity, we have to mention the secondary risk factors as well. Obese individuals usually have higher blood pressure than normal weight people. Hypertension is the number one risk factor for stroke.

Obese people often suffer from *sleep apnea*: during sleeping there are certain periods of decreased breathing, called "apneas". As a result of interrupted sleep, patients experience excessive daytime sleepiness and fatigue. Low oxygen levels and high blood pressure resulting from sleep apnea may further increase the risk of stroke in obese individuals. Abdominal obesity and body mass index higher than 30 are closely associated with sleep apnea.

Obese people have an increased risk of developing gallstones. The incidence of the disease is higher in women than in men. Estrogens increase cholesterol levels in bile and decrease gallbladder contractions, which may lead to the formation of gallstones.

Acid reflux is not necessarily a disease, but a physiological process that is also present in healthy people. The symptoms are considered pathological if they occur more than once a week. Frequently repeating refluxes of gastric acid from the stomach may erode the esophagus. *Gastroesophageal reflux disease* is closely associated with obesity. In the United States, 40% of the white population experience heartburn at least once a month.[5]

Obesity hypoventilation syndrome is a breathing disorder which may develop in obese people because of the body's impaired responsiveness to low O_2 and elevated CO_2 levels. Inadequate breathing may lead to serious complications such as pulmonary hypertension or leg edema. The severe form of the disease affecting extremely obese people is called *pickwickian syndrome*. Symptoms include irregular breathing, shortness of breath, fatigue, sleepiness during the day and right-sided heart failure.

Edema is the abnormal accumulation of fluid within the body. Fluid accumulation may occur in the lungs (pulmonary edema) or under the skin, typically in the legs or ankles. Severe obesity is often accompanied by excessive fluid retention. Severely obese patients may accumulate relatively large amounts of hidden fluid that can be easily overlooked. Edema is often associated with hypertension and heart failure.

In addition, one in five Americans has been diagnosed with arthritis. Arthritis is an inflammatory disease of the joints that often results in significant pain, swelling and stiffness. *Osteoarthritis* is the most common type of arthritis, that is directly linked to obesity. Obese people are at greater risk of developing the disease because of the increased stress on weight-bearing joints such as knees and hips.

Rheumatoid arthritis is an autoimmune disease in which the body's immune system attacks its own joint tissue. Fat cells produce inflammatory chemicals that can be associated with the development of the disease. *Gout* is the third common form of arthritis that is caused by the formation of uric acid crystals in the joints. Symptoms include painful attacks in the affected joints, typically in the big toe, knee or ankle. Obese people have ten times higher risk of developing gout.[6]

As mentioned previously, obesity is often accompanied by hypertension. In addition to being a considerable risk factor for life-threatening diseases such as heart disease or stroke, having a high blood pressure may also damage your vision. Elevated pressure in the eyes is associated with eye diseases such as cataract, glaucoma, and diabetic retinopathy.

THE PLAGUE

Obesity is a chronic metabolic disorder that affects every single organ of our body. As we have seen earlier, obesity is associated with a wide spectrum of life-threatening diseases. Type-2 diabetes and heart disease are the two most serious health conditions linked with obesity. Cardiovascular disease is the number one cause of death globally. Since the 20th century, obesity has claimed more lives than all wars, violent events and dictatorships combined, including World War I, World War II, all the genocides, civil wars, man-made famines and communism. Obesity deserves to be called the *plague of the 21st century.*

2

OBESITY IN DEVELOPING COUNTRIES

THE GLOBAL EPIDEMIC

In industrialized countries one third of the population is obese and another third is overweight. The phenomenon of obesity is not limited to the Western World alone; developing nations have been hit by the epidemic as well. In more than 70 countries, obesity rates have doubled since 1980 and *body mass indexes* continue to rise among every nation[7](see Figure 2.1). There are just a few places in the world where the number of obese people is the same as it was 40 years ago.

If you made a quick survey and asked people what the fattest country in the world is, you would probably have answers like "The United States" or a country in Europe. You may be surprised, but not Americans or Europeans are the champions of obesity. There is a tiny little island in the Pacific Ocean roughly 3,000 kilometers away from Australia and 10,000 kilometers from Mexico. The place is called *Nauru.* Here live the heaviest people on the earth. Seven out of every eight Nauruans are overweight and 61% of the population is obese.[8] As a result of obesity, Nauru has one of the highest prevalence rates of diabetes in the world. Over 42% of elderly people have been diagnosed with diabetes.[9] These statistics are outnumbered by one minority group only: the *Pima* Indians living on the Gila River Reservation in Arizona. Nauru, with its 11,000 residents, is the world's third smallest country behind Vatican City and Monaco. Phosphate was discovered on the island a century ago, and the exploitation of the reserves began shortly after that. Over the course of the following decades, the mining industry became so prosperous, that by the 1980s, Nauru had the highest GDP per capita in the world. In 1982, *The New York Times* called this miniature country "World's richest little isle". However, after the mineral deposits were exhausted, there

Body Mass Index, Men

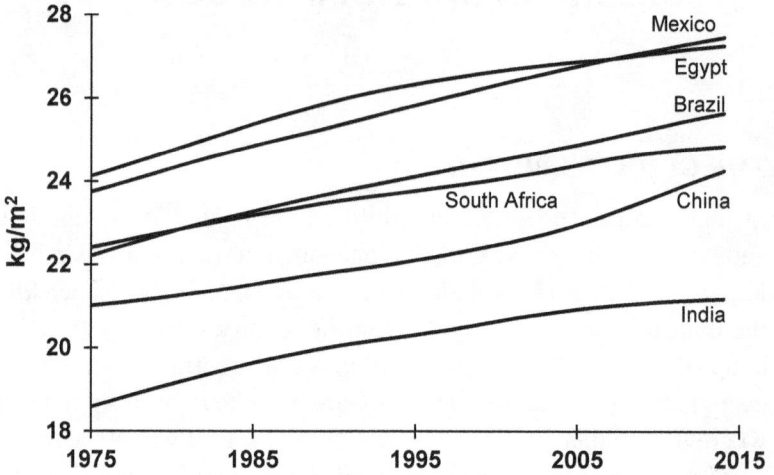

Body Mass Index, Women

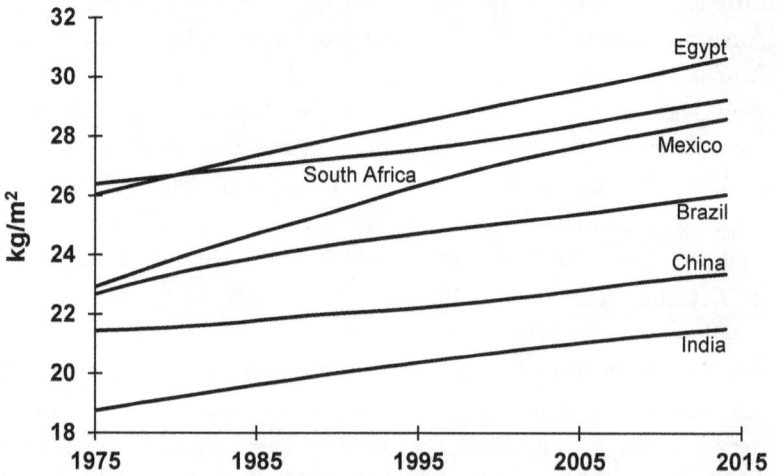

Figure 2.1. Change in body mass index between 1975-2014

was nothing left for the mining industry, just the abandoned phosphate plants and poverty. Due to the environmental catastrophe caused by phosphate mining, the whole island became uninhabitable, except for a narrow ring around the shoreline. The unemployment rate is estimated to be 90%. The former treasure island, which was once the richest country in the world, has become the fattest and sickest country in the world. As we will see in a later chapter of this book, obesity and poverty go together, just like French fries and ketchup at McDonald's.

The obesity epidemic originated in the United States, then swept across Europe, and by now it has become a serious threat to the health of the population even in the poorest countries of the world. Some of these regions suffered from malnutrition half a century ago, and today they struggle with obesity. How is all that possible? There are many explanations.

First of all, obesity is a *civilization disease*. Napoleon's physician, *Stanislas Tanchou* made a remarkable discovery: cancer was virtually non-existent in primitive cultures. Tanchou used to say that "Cancer, like insanity increases with civilization". If Dr. Tanchou lived in the 21st century, he would probably conclude that "Obesity, like insanity increases with civilization". Obesity has a noticeably higher prevalence rate in big urban centers compared with rural areas where people still live a traditional lifestyle. City dwellers tend to be physically less active; they use labor saving devices, motorized transport, and their westernized diet contains appreciable amounts refined carbohydrates.

CHINESE STUDIES

Traditionally, Chinese were considered to be very thin people. In today's China however, this is not necessarily true. One out of every three Chinese citizens is overweight and 6% of the population is obese.[8] Although these statistics are far better than U.S. obesity rates, we should keep in mind that the phenomenon of obesity was basically unknown in 1970s' China. Over the course of the last decades, China has experienced an extremely rapid pace of wealth accumulation. With this unprecedented economic growth, inequalities within the country are also rising faster than anywhere else. China's urban population benefits disproportionately more from the wealth redistribution than the residents of rural areas. Urban Chinese live a more sedentary lifestyle and they are more likely to consume Western food containing excessive amounts of refined carbohydrates, especially sugar, which was not a part of the traditional Chinese diet. Since the 1960s, the sugar production per capita in China has tripled and wheat is getting more common (see Figure 2.2). As a result of the increasing popularity of the Western lifestyle, the Chinese have gotten more obese than ever before and they keep on growing heavier every single year (see Figure 2.3).

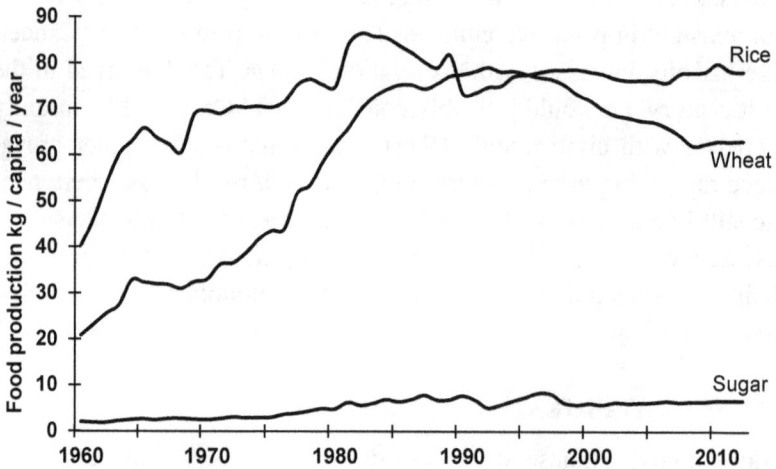

Figure 2.2. Rice, wheat and sugar production in China

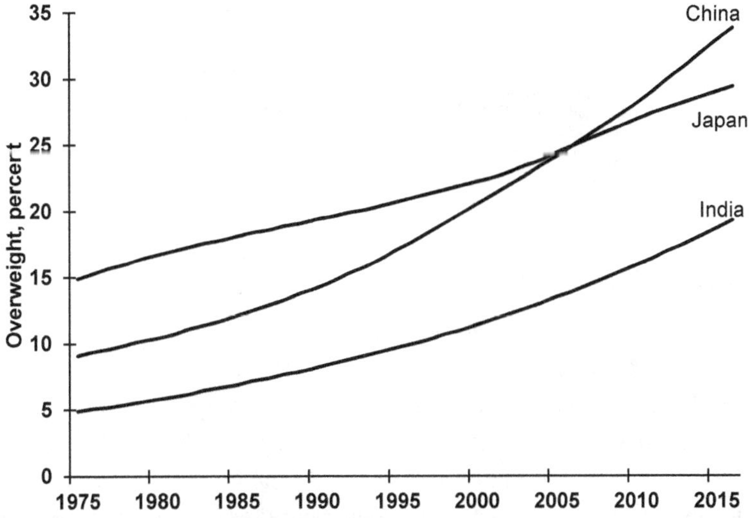

Figure 2.3. The myth that China is the thinnest nation is not true. India has always been leaner than China. Recently, the Japanese were outweighed by the Chinese. The chart shows the percentage of overweight people in the three countries.

3

OBESITY AND ETHNICITY

AMERICAN STUDIES

Obesity has become a nationwide epidemic in the United States. Over the past few decades, the number of obese adults has more than doubled. In this chapter, we will examine the impact of the obesity epidemic on the two largest minority groups in the United States. Although the whole country is affected by the epidemic, the increase in the prevalence of obesity has been remarkably higher among the Black and Mexican populations compared to any other groups.

Based on the *National Health and Nutrition Examination Survey* data, one out of every three White adults is obese.[10] Asians are the thinnest: only one tenth of the Asian population falls into the obese category. The highest prevalence rate of obesity was found among the Black population (48%), followed by Hispanic adults (42 %) (see Figure 3.1). These statistics include the number of obese individuals only, whose *body mass index* is 30 or higher. An additional third of Americans, whose BMI is between 25 and 30, is classified as overweight; and the final third of the population is a normal body weight. The most striking difference in the prevalence of obesity was found between Asian and Black women, who are 5 times more likely to be obese.

There are many possible explanations for the interracial inequalities in obesity rates. For example, low income levels are directly correlated to obesity. Families living under the poverty line can not afford to purchase nutritious food items; parents and children are more likely to buy energy-dense, highly processed food. Families who live in minority and low-income neighborhoods may have limited access to supermarkets and fresh produce. Citizens living in impoverished areas don't have easy access to parks and recreation

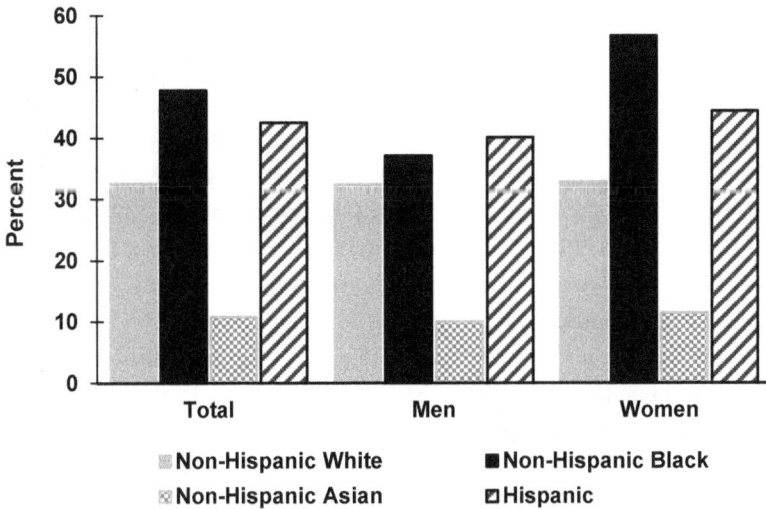

Figure 3.1. Prevalence of obesity in the USA, by sex and ethnicity

facilities. As a result, they also tend to be physically less active. A sedentary lifestyle is one of the main contributory factors to the development of obesity and many chronic diseases.

Minority groups are the primary targets of junk food companies and restaurants. In their advertising campaigns, those businesses often hire African-American sport celebrities for their commercials specifically targeting a Black audience. On average, Black children see twice as many food commercials compared to White children, and they will be less likely to make healthy food choices later in their lives.[11]

The Hispanic population in the United States is the nation's largest minority group. The high prevalence rate of obesity is a growing concern throughout the Hispanic communities of America. An astonishing 81 % of the Mexican American adult population is overweight or obese.[12] During the past few decades, the number of overweight adults has been rising continuously; three decades earlier "only" two thirds of Mexican Americans fell into the overweight category. At the same time, the percentage of obese Mexican-American children grew from 13% to 23%. The increasing popularity of junk food and sweetened beverages are closely related to today's obesity epidemic.

According to *Salud America*, Latino kids consume more sugar in the form of soda, fruit drinks and flavored milk than an average American child.[13] Parents feed their children with sweetened beverages from their early infancy to their late teens. About 74% of Latinos have consumed sugary drinks by the age of two, compared to 45% of non-Latino Whites. Food companies pay special attention to children and teenagers as their future customers when advertising their products. Popular soccer athletes and Latino music celebrities often appear on food commercials.

There is another possible explanation for the inequality in obesity rates between different ethnic groups. Social norms regarding ideal body weight may differ significantly among various cultures. An interesting study was conducted on a representative sample of 389 White, Hispanic, and Black women.[14] A self-image assessment was done, to find out how satisfied women are with their body weight. To measure the participants' satisfaction level, researchers introduced a new term called *"body image discrepancy"* (BD), which was compared to the women's actual body mass index. Among different racial groups there was no difference in the subjects' satisfaction level. White women however, experienced BD at a much lower body mass index (BMI=24.6), which is below the cutoff point of the overweight category (BMI=25). In contrast, Hispanic and Black women reported BD at a much higher body mass index (BMI of 28.5 and 29.2, respectively). In other words, Black women experience less social pressure to be thin, mostly because Black men tend to prefer larger body sizes in female partners.

In addition to these previously mentioned factors, the ethnic composition of the neighborhood where an individual lives also plays an important role in the development of obesity. For example, those who live in Chinatown, where Asian stores are plentiful, and restaurants with more natural food choices are available, tend to purchase less processed food. Statistical data supports the fact that White people living in predominantly Asian neighborhoods are less likely to be obese.[15]

CANADIAN STUDIES

Canada has been a multicultural country for a very long period of time. Canada's diverse population provides a great opportunity to study the differences in the prevalence of obesity among groups of different people with various ethnic backgrounds. Because of its proximity to the USA, both countries show many common features. However, Canada has significantly lower adult obesity prevalence rates than the United States.

The following brief overview is based on the information from the *Canadian Community Health Surveys* conducted by *Statistics Canada*.[16] Over 86,000 individuals participated in the study, who were classified based on their ethnic background into the following categories: White, Chinese, South Asian, Black, Filipino, Latin American, Southeast Asian, Arab, West Asian, Japanese, Korean, Aboriginal and other. Researchers found that the thinnest people in Canada are those of East / Southeast Asian origin with an obesity prevalence rate of 3%. About 17% of the White population and 28% of the Aboriginals were found to be obese. Overall, the prevalence of obesity in Canada is apparently lower than in the United States. Remarkably, recent immigrants tend to be significantly leaner than those who were born in Canada. The difference between the two groups however, disappears over time.

BRITISH STUDIES

The prevalence of obesity in the UK, as in every single industrialized country, has been steadily increasing over the last few decades. The *Health Survey for England* is an annual report on the overall health of the British population. The health status of certain minority groups was the focus of the 2004 survey[17], with special regards to cardiovascular disease. Based on the 2001 census data, 92% of the UK population is White, and the remaining 8% belong to one of the minority groups. In 2004, the body mass index, waist-to-hip ratio and waist circumference data were analyzed among the following ethnic groups: Black Caribbean, Black African, Indian, Pakistani, Bangladeshi, Chinese, Irish and also for the general population. Figure 3.2

shows the percentage of obese people based on BMI data, within six ethnic groups. As for the prevalence of obesity, the study shows a remarkable difference between Black African men and women: the likelihood of obesity for women is twice as high as for men. Interestingly, Black African men are less obese, and Black African women are more obese than Black Caribbeans. Like in the previous two studies, Chinese are the thinnest among the eight ethnic groups. The obesity rate of the White population was found to be similar to the Canadian survey data.

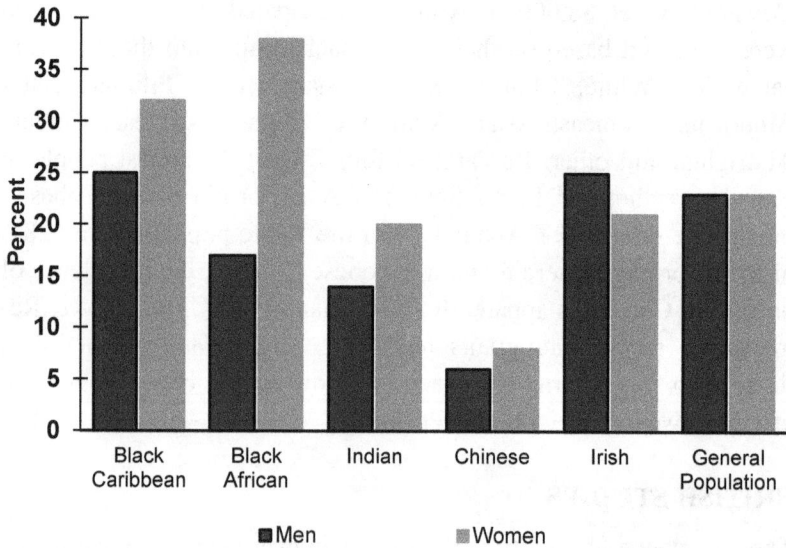

Figure 3.2. Prevalence of obesity in the UK, by sex and ethnicity

4

CHILDHOOD OBESITY

ALARMING RATES OF CHILDHOOD OBESITY

In the 21st century, the epidemic of obesity is no longer limited to adults. The number of the obese and overweight is rising at an alarming rate among children and adolescents. Since the 1970s, the prevalence of childhood obesity has more than tripled. In 2014, 20.5% of adolescents were found to be obese: roughly one in every five kids. This is the national average. However, children belonging to certain minority groups tend to be even more obese, as we saw in the previous chapter.

For adults, *body mass index* (BMI) is the most widely used and accepted measure of obesity. For children however, a different method was developed since their BMI continuously changes. A child's weight status is determined by an age-specific percentile of BMI. Overweight is defined as BMI at or above the 85th percentile of a reference population. In plain language, a child is called overweight if he / she weighs more than 85% of the other children in the same age group. Children, who are heavier than 95% of the other children in their age group are considered to be obese.

HISTORIC OVERVIEW

Childhood obesity is not new a phenomenon. Since the Middle Ages and the Renaissance, famous painters very often depicted obese men, women and children. In those days, obesity wasn't considered a chronic disease, but rather a sign of wealth. *Peter Paul Rubens*, who lived four centuries ago, painted hundreds, if not thousands of obese characters among his known 1,400 works. If we oversimplify Rubens' art, his paintings can be put into two categories: those with normal weight and those with obese people. The young boy on his famous painting *Bacchus* definitely would fall into the 95th percentile of the reference population. Another example is Juan Carreño de Miranda, a Spanish painter of the Baroque period, who portrays a severely obese 6 year old girl known as *La Monstrua Vestida*, or *The Dressed Monster*; a possible case of Prader-Willi syndrome. Upon seeing the painting in Madrid, *Dr. Andrea Prader*, who first described the disease, immediately recognized the features of Prader-Willi syndrome of the 6-year-old girl.

Apart from a few extreme cases, childhood obesity was very rare until the 20th century. Things first started to change a hundred years ago around the major urban centers of the United states. When the German physician *Hilde Bruch*, an expert on eating disorders, arrived in New York City in 1934, she noticed the huge number of really obese children not only in the clinics, but also on the streets, subways and in schools. However, with the exception of a few metropolitan areas, childhood obesity was virtually non-existent in the rest of the world, even including the United States.

A paper was published on the history of childhood obesity in the U.S.[18] There is very limited data available for the period preceding the first national survey in 1963. Using body mass index data from *The Fels Longitudinal Study,* researchers analyzed the prevalence rate of childhood obesity. Representative samples were collected in Dayton, Ohio from the time period spanning between 1930 and 1993. Over six decades, the prevalence of obesity rose from 0% to 14% among boys and from 2% to 12% among girls. During the next two decades the obesity rate climbed even higher, reaching the 20% mark.

FAILED ATTEMPTS TO STOP THE EPIDEMIC

Health authorities, physicians, dieticians, teachers and parents have teamed up many times and made gigantic efforts to stop the childhood obesity epidemic. However, every single attempt has failed over the last few decades. Kids just keep getting heavier each year. Readers may ask the question: Why are all childhood prevention programs destined to fail? The answer is very simple: for the same reason that adults fail. The whole concept of how we look at the phenomenon of obesity is totally wrong. According to the *World Health*

Organization's definition: "The fundamental cause of obesity and overweight is an energy imbalance between calories consumed and calories expended." This approach is basically the same as the classic *Calories In, Calories Out* model that has been the most widely-accepted view since the second half of the 20th century. With the practical application of this theory, we are just getting heavier and heavier, year after year. The *Calories In, Calories Out* chapter of this book gives a detailed explanation on the topic of why *calorie counting* does not work in the long run.

We will see in the *Hormonal Obesity* chapter, that Obesity and type-2 diabetes have the same underlying cause. To address the risk factors for diabetes in middle school-aged children, a large-scale study was conducted with the participation of over six thousand grade 6 to 8 students. The program is known as the *HEALTHY* study.[19] The main objectives included:

- Increasing the students' physical activity level up to 225 minutes in every two weeks
- Educating students, parents and teachers about healthy food choices
- A "TV turnoff" challenge and a 7 hour per week TV budget
- Lower the fat content of food served in school
- Reduce the energy content of snack food to <200 kcal
- Least 2 servings of fruit and/or vegetables
- Eliminate fat milk and added sugar beverages
- Least 2 servings of grain-based foods and/or legumes

Students were followed from the baseline (6th grade) until the end of the study (8th grade). At the beginning of the program, about half of the students were overweight or obese. Surprisingly, at the end, there was no difference in obesity rates between those students who participated in the program and those who didn't. In both groups, 45% of the students were in the overweight or obese category. Unfortunately, the program turned out to be a complete failure. It looks like the worldwide childhood obesity epidemic can not be stopped by measures like a "TV turnoff challenge" or two daily servings of fruits or vegetables. Why?

PARTIAL RESULTS

Besides the *HEALTHY* Study, there were other attempts as well to limit the time children spend watching television. Sitting for long hours in the front of the screen every day, interferes with our health several ways: by replacing outdoor activities with our favorite TV programs, snacking while watching shows and buying more junk food as a result of commercials. With the participation of 192 third and fourth grade students, researchers examined the relationship between the time spent watching television, playing video games and obesity[20]. Following a "TV turnoff" challenge, children were given a 7-hour-per-week TV budget. By the end of the 7-month study, the body mass index of the participants decreased by 0.45 and their waist circumference by 2.3 cm. Although the results were called statistically significant, this experiment had just a minimal, hardly noticeable impact on obesity.

The fattening effect of sugar-sweetened beverages has been well-known for decades. A study was done with 224 participating overweight and obese adolescents who regularly consumed large amounts of pop and fruit juices.[21] Those, who reduced their sugary drink consumption to near zero, experienced a minor change in their BMI (-0.57) after a year. However, by the end of the second year, the differences slowly disappeared, as the participants gradually returned to their old habit of drinking sugar-sweetened beverages. Interestingly, those of Hispanic ethnicity within the group achieved a significant weight loss: 6.4 kg by the end of the first year and 8.8 kg by the end of the second year.

OBESE BABIES

As we saw earlier, the number of obese school-aged children and adolescents has been continuously growing since the 1970s. On the other hand, obesity in early childhood is a relatively new phenomenon. A study was done with the participation of over 120,000 children aged 0 to 6 years. Researchers examined how the number of obese and overweight children changed during the period between 1980 and 2001.[22] Over two decades, obesity largely increased in every single age group. The most striking difference was found among children between 24 and 36 months. In this group, the number of obese children has doubled in just 21 years (see Figure 4.1). At a very early age, children become trained to love super-sweet flavors. Breast milk contains 7% of carbohydrates, most of it in the form of *lactose*. It should be noted that the sweetness of lactose is not even close to other sugars; for example, sucrose (table sugar) is 6 times sweeter than lactose. Many baby formula manufacturers – especially those in the United States – add sucrose to their products to make them tastier for babies. They take advantage of a loophole in the food labeling regulations: it is not mandatory to show the sugar content of infant formulas. The well-known television station *NBC 5 Chicago* hired an independent laboratory to analyze the sugar content of seven popular infant formulas.[23] Experts found up to 13.5 grams of sugar per serving in the provided samples. Due to the fattening effect of table sugar, European authorities banned sucrose from baby formulas in 2009. In contrast, manufacturers argue that sugar is nutritious,

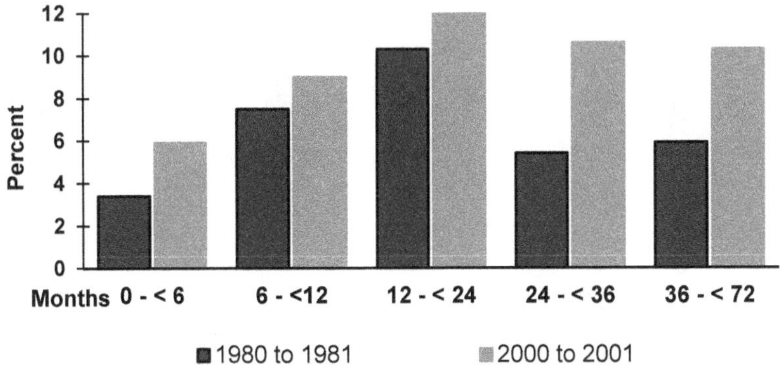

Figure 4.1. Obesity in early childhood in different age groups

easily digestible, and plays an important role in the development of children. Only the second one of the above statements is correct: sugar is easily digestible. As for the rest, there is no scientific evidence to prove those claims.

Statistics from the *Feeding Infants and Toddlers Study* show that an average child, between 2 and 4 years in the United States, consumes 221 kcal from sweets and snacks and an additional 72 kcal from sugary juices every day.[24] Over time, as the child grows, so does his / her sugar intake. A study was done to determine the sugar content of infant formulas, baby foods and grocery items prepared for children.[25] Researchers found that on average 38% of the energy content of baby foods comes from sugar, but certain products have an even higher sugar content. In other words, baby food is not much better than adult's junk food; both are composed of excessive amounts of highly concentrated refined carbohydrates. In *Part II* of this book, we will discuss in depth the fattening effects of carbohydrates.

5

POVERTY AND OBESITY

WHY ARE POOR PEOPLE MORE LIKELY TO BE OBESE?

Traditionally, obesity has been associated with wealth and affluence. High-income countries usually have greater rates of obesity than middle and low-income countries. Interestingly, if we examine the prevalence of obesity within the United States or any other industrialized country, we will see the opposite trend. Those who live in poverty are more likely to be obese than affluent people. In the United States, 46 million people live under the poverty line: one out of every six citizens. This is the highest number in more than 50 years.

In a review of 3,139 counties in the U.S., a very close association was found between poverty and obesity. Counties with high poverty rates (>35%) , have a 145% greater prevalence of obesity.[26] There are millions of food insecure people throughout the United States. However, food insecurity in America substantially differs from developing countries. While the concerned Third World countries suffer from malnutrition as a result of food scarcity, the United States has a *qualitative* rather than *quantitative* food shortage. Low-income families cannot afford to buy healthy food items; parents and children are more likely to buy energy-dense, highly-processed food. Citizens living in impoverished neighborhoods have limited access to supermarkets and fresh produce. Such areas are often called *food deserts*.

Energy density of foods is a function of their water content. Generally speaking, the less energy-dense foods are heavily hydrated, and the energy-dense foods are dry, containing high amounts of sugar, starch and fat. The energy density of foods is measured in MJ/kg (1 kilogram food's energy content in megajoules). For example, wheat flour is an energy-packed food item with an energy density of 15.2 MJ/kg or sugar with 16.2 MJ/kg. On the other hand, cauliflower is a low energy-density food, only 1 MJ/kg. Energy-dense foods, for example wheat, corn, rice and sugar are heavily subsidized by governments. As a result, these items are relatively inexpensive; their $/calorie cost is the lowest of all. Therefore, cheap food items high in refined carbohydrates are the only available choice for impoverished families. Such foods are the most fattening ones. The consumption of unhealthy food is one of the main contributing factors to today's obesity epidemic.

In addition to bad dietary habits, in the development of obesity, physical inactivity plays an important role as well. Citizens living in impoverished areas tend to be physically less active; this can be partially explained by their limited access to parks and recreational facilities, as well as higher unemployment rates.

Poverty and obesity go hand in hand. There was an interesting picture posted on Wikipedia.[27] It was of a severely obese man standing in the line of a *soup kitchen*; waiting to be served a free lunch in a place that provides food for the poor. Doesn't it seem   illogical?

6

THE FATTEST MEN THAT EVER LIVED

THE LIFE OF ROBERT EARL HUGHES

Robert Earl Hughes (1926-1958) during his very short life got listed in *The Guinness Book of World Records* as the heaviest human being in the history (Figure 6.1). After he was born, his family moved to a farm near *Fishhook*, Illinois. Fishhook is so small, that it can't even be found on the map. The town has a general store, two churches, and a one-room schoolhouse.

When Robert Earl Hughes was born, he weighed just a little bit more than normal. Hughes' sister-in-law says that at the age of 6 months he had *whooping cough* and "ruptured the thyroid gland". We don't know exactly what happened, but from that point on, Hughes started gaining weight and he never stopped. At the age of ten he weighed 378 pounds[28]. A doctor who examined Robert Earl, told his parents that they should not expect that their son would live longer than 15 years because the boy's heart couldn't stand such stress.

Robert Earl was a very talented child, and had an excellent memory. If he read something or met someone, he would remember forever. He was a very kind and happy person who had many friends. In the eyes of his classmates, Robert Earl didn't appear any different, just a little bit bigger.

As Robert Earl grew heavier, his daily walk from home to the one room school building became more and more challenging. One day, on his way back from school Robert Earl fell into a muddy ditch. It took a tractor, and several men with belts to pull him out of the mud. At the end of seventh grade, he quit school and stayed at home to help his mother. At the age of 16, the boy weighed 600 pounds and by the time he turned 20 he was over 700 pounds. As the word spread in the surrounding counties about the fat boy, visitors started to flock to Fishhook to see the attraction. Later, he appeared at carnivals and fairs. People would line up to pay 25 cents for admission and to buy photographs of the 700-pound man. Hughes' new business turned out to be very profitable, and he was making more money than anyone in his family ever had. At the end of the Baylis Fall Festival, he grossed $240 ($2,000 in today's dollars).

In 1956, Hughes already weighed 1,041 pounds. In his custom built van, he was touring in the South, East, and Midwest. One day he was approached by a man, offering him the opportunity of his lifetime: to appear on New York's biggest television show, a $40,000 paycheck plus airfare and expenses. There was a problem however: no passenger airline could fly the 1,041-pound Robert Earl Hughes to New York. Finally with special permission from the Civil Aeronautics Board, he was taken by a freight carrier. The ambulance took him to the airport and he was lifted into the airplane by a crane. On his New York appearance, Hughes had to wear the world's biggest Santa Claus suit. Hundreds of photos were taken of the heaviest Santa ever. However, shortly after that, the promoter was gone. Hughes suddenly realized that he fell victim to a scam: no money, no television show. Robert Earl Hughes got stuck in New York without a place to stay or a ticket back home. Finally, he managed to return home with the help of the Salvation Army.

During the last two years of his life, Hughes was traveling throughout the country with his brother and his sister-in-law. At that time, walking was nearly impossible for the 31-year-old man. In 1958, during his Midwest tour the 32-year-old Hughes contracted measles. A few days after hospitalization, Robert Earl Hughes died from congestive heart failure.

OTHER HEAVY PEOPLE

Over the course of six decades following the death of Robert Earl Hughes, even more obese people came and took his title of the world's heaviest man. *Wikipedia* lists ten individuals who weighed even more than Hughes did. According to the *Guinness Book of World Records* the heaviest person in medical history was *Jon Brower Minnoch* (1941–1983). Minnoch suffered from obesity since

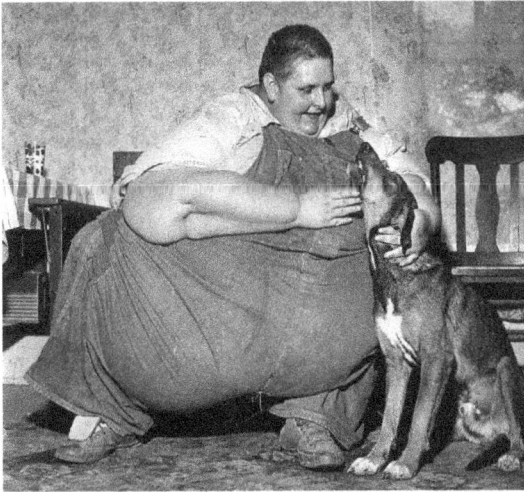

Figure 6.1. Robert Earl Hughes

his childhood. At age 12, his weight was 291 pounds and by 22 he was 392 pounds. He was 185 cm (6 ft 1 in) tall. At his peak, he weighed approximately 1,400 lb or 635 kilograms. His weight was only an estimate because his extreme size and the lack of mobility prevented the use of a scale. Based on his estimated weight, his *body mass index* was about 185 kg/m². The *World Health Organization* classifies BMI>30 as *obese* and BMI>35 as *severely obese*. The highest existing obesity class is BMI>60. Minnoch's BMI was even three times higher than that.

In 1978, he married his 110-pound wife Jeannette; they broke the record for the greatest difference in weight between spouses. Later, Jon and Jeannette had two children. The same year he got married, Minnoch was diagnosed with generalized edema, a medical condition of abnormally large fluid accumulation in the body. He was admitted to the University of Washington Medical Center in Seattle.

The transportation of Minnoch was not an easy task. Moving the 1400-pound man from his home to the ferry boat and to the hospital took a dozen firemen and a custom made stretcher. In the hospital, he was laid on two beds pushed together. It took 13 people to roll him over for linen changes. Minnoch was put on a very strict diet drastically limiting his energy intake to 1,200 calories per day. Sixteen months later, when he was discharged from the hospital, Minnoch weighed 476 pounds "only". He lost 924 pounds in total.

Jon Brower Minnoch was an extraordinary man who broke three world records:

- Heaviest human being ever lived
- The greatest weight difference between spouses
- Achieved the largest human weight loss ever documented

A year later as his edema worsened, he started gaining weight again and was readmitted to the hospital. Since his condition was incurable, he decided to discontinue the treatment and died at the age of 41.

PART

TWO

WHAT CAUSES OBESITY

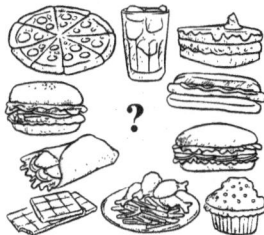

PART

TWO

WHAT CAUSES OBESITY

7

STORY OF THE PIMA INDIANS

WHAT CAN WE LEARN FROM THEM?

Every single considerable scientific work written on the topic of obesity mentions the case of the *Pima Indians*. The Pima people are a group of Native Americans living in Central and Southern Arizona and in the Mexican state of Sonora. Today, Pima Indians have the highest incidence of obesity and diabetes in North America. In the United States, almost two thirds of the Pima men and three quarters of the women were found to be obese.[29] The average *body mass index* (BMI) of the entire Pima population in Arizona was well over 30.[30] According to the WHO, individuals with a BMI above 30 are considered to be obese. As a result of the obesity epidemic, one of the highest prevalence rates of type-2 diabetes in the world was found among the Pima, living on the Gila River Indian Reservation in Arizona. Nearly 69% of the women aged 55 to 64 were diabetic.[31] These numbers are 9 times higher than the national average for Caucasians and 4 times higher than other Native American people. Chronic liver disease and kidney failure resulting from diabetes are also common problems among the Pima population in Arizona. Although Native Americans have the longest life expectancy in the United States (88 years for women and 84 years for men), Indians living in Arizona are expected to die at the age of 60.

Pima Indians haven't always been among the ethnic groups in the United States considered in poor health. In 1846, when the United States Army passed through Pima lands, the assistant surgeon of the battalion, John Strother Griffin, described the Pima in his diary as "sprightly good-tempered fellows". Griffin also says "These people seem to enjoy fine health". He made no mention of obesity, diabetes, kidney or liver disease.

The Pima Indians have always been a friendly, peaceful nation. They used to be farmers and hunter-gatherers who were organized into two social groups called the *Red Ants* and the *White Ants*. Centuries ago on the fertile lands of the Gila valley the Pima built a intricate irrigation system. The men's job was clearing the land, digging the canals and planting the crops. All these tasks required hard physical labor, considering the fact that the Native Americans did not traditionally use draft animals such as horses or oxen. The women harvested the crops, carried the products, did the house work, wove their clothing and made baskets. The Pima Indians were brilliant agriculturists. The typical Pima diet consisted of a wide array of plant-based foods such as wheat, corn, different legumes (such as lentils, chickpeas, tepary beans and lima beans), amaranth, chia seeds, velvet mesquite, screwbean mesquite, indianwheat, pepper, tomato, gourd, sorghum, cotton seed, agave, mushrooms, acorns, figs, apricots, peaches, elderberries, watermelon, and the fruit of edible cactus species. Cattle and poultry was kept for meat; occasionally game, fish and clams from the Gila river were added to their menu.

After 1849, when the California gold rush began, tens of thousands of prospectors traveled through Pima lands, following the Gila route. In those days, Pima people still lived in prosperity. Food was so abundant that they produced not only enough for themselves but also supplied the travelers with everything they needed. During the following decades however, as Anglo-Americans began settling in large numbers in the Gila Valley, the age of affluence of the Pima came to an end. The new settlers took their land from the Indians and they were forced onto reservations. In the 1870s and 1880s, as non-Native farmers diverted the river, the farming of the Pima Indians was largely wiped out. Between 1880 and 1920 the Pima faced mass famine and starvation. This is the time when the federal government intervened by handing out large amounts of cheap processed food.

During the early 20th century, two prominent anthropologists began to study the Pima Indians. The first one was Frank Russell from Harvard University. In his 1908 book, Russell wrote about the Pima: "They are noticeably heavier than individuals belonging to the tribes on the Colorado plateau" ... "Many old persons exhibit a degree of obesity that is in striking contrast with the tall and sinewy Indian conventionalized in popular thought".[32]From the book, a photograph of a severely obese elderly woman became famous as *"Fat Louisa"*. Russell made an astonishing discovery more than a century ago: he realized that some elements of their diet made them noticeably fatter than other Indians. "Certain articles of their diet appear to be markedly flesh producing".

In the same year, Aleš Hrdlička of Smithsonian Institution published a book entitled: *Physiological and Medical Observations Among the Indians of Southwestern United States and Northern Mexico*. Hrdlička encountered overweight Indians virtually in every tribe, however the severely obese ones were typically women and those who lived on reservations. He noted that "Especially well-nourished individuals, females and also males, occur in every tribe and at all ages, but real obesity is found almost exclusively among the Indians on reservations" ... "Among the Pima it is largely, but not exclusively, the women who grow very stout". Interestingly, obesity was rare among the Pueblo Indians, who had had sedentary habits since ancient times.

In the second half of the 19th century as the non-Native settlers gradually displaced the Indians, the Pima had to leave their land and were forced to live on reservations designated by the federal government. In the new environment, the Pima had to give up their traditional lifestyle. Of course, these significant changes had an enormous impact on their dietary habits as well. The former hunter-gatherers and farmers facing starvation, and now had to rely on the government rationing system. Cheap processed food was distributed among the Indians by the tons. New trading posts appeared on the reservations where the white man's food was sold exclusively. Sugar, wheat, flour and lard became regular commodities. Native Americans discovered a new kind of cooking: grease frying. The recipe of the "authentic" *Indian fry bread* was born. As the newly introduced food items became more and more popular, the traditional Pima foods were gradually forgotten. *A.M. Rea*, another researcher, listed more than 50 neglected plant species which was be an important part of the Pima diet for centuries.[33] The list of discarded plant products include our recently rediscovered super-health food, the chia seed, which is rich in omega-3 fatty acids, fiber, protein, minerals and vitamins. Soluble dietary fiber containing *psyllium* products that are marketed under several brand names, are used in the prevention and treatment of various ailments and conditions, and can be found on the shelves of virtually every pharmacy and health store. Psyllium is also known as *indianwheat* and used to be a part of the traditional Pima diet until the 20th century.

Indians who were farming at the edge of the desert for centuries were taught by government farm advisors how to replace their self sustaining, organic farming techniques with corporate models. As a result of such enforced modernization, many of the wild food plants from the flood plains became unavailable. The ancient desert crop varieties were neglected and by the second half of the 20th century, most of the traditional foods fell from common use. During the last century their overall nutritional quality continuously declined. Today, the diet of a typical Pima Indian is even poorer in quality than that of the general American population. What can we learn from the Pima? Highly processed foods based on excessive amounts of refined carbohydrates combined with a physically inactive lifestyle and the separation from their natural environment turned the tall, lean Pima Indians into obese people suffering from all sorts of health conditions.

8

INHERITED OBESITY

THE FAT GENE MYTH

We tend to attribute our own and others' behavior to inborn biological causes. With the advancement of science, we have manufactured genetic explanations of why we continuously fail in changing the unchangeable. Genetic explanations for depression, alcoholism, drug addiction, intelligence, behavioral disorders or even criminality appear in newspaper headlines on a regular basis. Obesity is no exception. People often assume that since obesity "runs in their families", there is nothing to do about it.

If we take a closer look, obesity is a complex disorder, determined by an equation of various influences such as genetical, hormonal, environmental, neurological, behavioral, psychological and developmental factors. Although genetics is an important part of the equation, genes by themselves do not cause obesity (except for a few extremely rare cases).

Considering the fact that in industrialized countries nearly one third of the population is obese and the other third is in the overweight category, only a negligible portion of these people have a primary genetic cause for their weight problem. Leptin gene mutation is one of the possible causes of monogenic obesity. In these rare cases mutant genes terminate leptin production. Leptin is a hormone produced by fat cells that regulates the energy balance of our body by suppressing hunger. In leptin deficient patients, obesity can be easily reversed by leptin treatment. On the other hand, in certain individuals, in spite of high serum leptin levels, the hormone has no effect because of leptin receptor mutation. The phenomenon of obesity caused by the mutation of a single gene is very rare: only a few hundred cases were identified worldwide.

Prader-Willi syndrome is a genetic disorder characterized by chronic hunger, excessive eating, and life threatening obesity often accompanied with type-2 diabetes, as well as short stature, moderate intellectual impairment and learning disabilities. Prader-Willi syndrome occurs when a segment of the father's chromosome 15 is deleted or the individual has two copies of chromosome 15 from his or her mother instead of one copy from each parent. Prader-Willi syndrome is not inherited; it's a genetic error that occurs randomly during conception or early fetal development. Although Prader-Willi syndrome is the most common genetic cause of morbid obesity in children, it occurs only once in every 25,000 births. [4]

Except for such extremely rare cases, most of the time obesity is a result of the interaction of many different genes. There is no such thing as the "Fat Gene". Over 80 genes have been identified that are known to be associated with obesity, however each one alone plays just a modest role in the etiology of the disorder.

From time to time, newspapers come up with headlines like "Scientists discover how key gene makes people fat". This article in particular was published in *USA Today* on August 19, 2015, and the author claimed that the key gene associated with obesity was finally found. Although the article didn't say it, readers still had the impression that help is on its way and we don't need to worry anymore about dieting. In the near future, by taking the new miracle pill we can eat as much as we want–we don't even need to exercise–but still expect to be lean and healthy for life.

The cited article was referring to the *fat mass and obesity associated gene* (FTO), which is one the 80 potential obesity genes. The FTO gene regulates the body's energy expenditure and the maturing of fat cells. The gene prevents the conversion of fat storing white adipocytes to heat producing beige adipocytes. In experimental animals, inactivation of the gene reduced body weight without a change in physical activity or appetite. In Europe, a study was conducted with the participation of over 38,000 subjects. Researchers found a positive association between obesity and the presence of the FTO gene. Compared to normal subjects, those individuals carrying the gene weighed 3 kg more on average and the odds of obesity increased 1.67 times.[34]

The article from *USA Today* said that: "Independent experts praised the discovery". According to the researchers, all it takes is a 3 kg (6.6 lb) difference in body weight to determine what makes you thin or obese? Well, if we talked about 30 kg, it would definitely make sense. Obviously, three kilograms is next to nothing. "Independent experts" call a 3 kg difference a "big deal". Most scientists would agree that a 3 kg variance in body weight is insignificant; your weight can fluctuate by that amount in a single day.

TWIN AND ADOPTION STUDIES

The contribution of genetic factors related to obesity is estimated by *Hernandez* to be between 40 and 70 percent.[35] Besides genetics, there is a wide range of environmental factors that play an important role in the pathogenesis of obesity. The consumption of excessive amounts of refined carbohydrates is the first factor. If you take time to carefully study the labels of the foods we consume on a daily basis, you will be shocked to realize that sugar is added to almost every single food item. People eat more fast food than ever before, and restaurants tend to supersize their meals. Junk food is easily accessible everywhere through vending machines set up in schools, hospitals, train stations, sports and community events etc.

Physical activity level is another important environmental factor as well. Compared to our grandparents' generation we are physically less active. Instead of outdoor activities, we spend more time in the front of the screens of our computers, televisions, video games and smartphones.

There is no doubt about the important role of genetics in the development of obesity. Until today, however there is no consensus among researchers on the original question of how much variation is explained by genetic factors alone. The previously-cited article estimated the impact of genetics on our body weight to be in the range of 40 to 70 percent, which at first sight seems reasonable. However, if we dig a little bit deeper, we will come across a large amount of conflicting data.

Adoption studies and *twin studies* are two classic methods to determine the effects of genetic factors in the pathogenesis of obesity. The objective of *adoption studies* is to estimate the significance of culture versus genes in the transmission of obesity by comparing adoptees to their adoptive parents and children to their biological parents. In *twin studies*, the strength of genetic factors is estimated by comparing the degree of obesity between twin pairs living in separate environments.

In our model, regarding the genes' role in the development of obesity, the original 40-70% window needs to be expanded. *Maes et al.* performed a meta-analysis on the familial resemblance of body mass index, based on the results of *adoption studies* and *twin studies*.[36] Researchers analyzed body weight data obtained from more than 25,000 twin pairs and 50,000 biological and adoptive family members. *Maes* found that 50 to 90 percent of the variance in obesity between twin pairs can be explained by genetic factors alone. Results from examining the *body mass index* of 7,000 Finnish twin pairs showed that as we get older, the role of genetics becomes less important and the role of the environment becomes more influential in the development of obesity. Higher heritabilities were also reported for men compared to women.

On the other hand, in *adoption studies,* the heritability of obesity was found to be much weaker. It was in the range of 20 to 60% in parent-child relations. In most countries, data on biological parents of adoptees is confidential and therefore is not easily accessible for researchers. One exception is the Danish Adoption Register. *Albert J. Stunkard* conducted a study on 540 adult Danish adoptees.[37] He was examining the mechanisms of how genetics and environmental factors can affect obesity. Based on weight and height data available from the Register, Stunkard put the subjects into four weight groups: obese, overweight, normal weight, and thin. He found a strong correlation between the weight categories of the adoptees and their biological parents. On the contrary, there was no apparent correlation between the weight of adoptees and their adoptive parents. In other words, if Stunkard was right, then the environment, where adopted children are raised has no influence on their weight. The destiny of a child is written in his / her genes. If you were born to be obese you will become obese. If you were born to be thin, you can eat as much as you want and you will stay thin for your entire life. Although Albert J. Stunkard is one of the most frequently cited authors specialized in the genetics of obesity: in his work he overemphasized the role of genetic factors in the development of obesity. In the previously mentioned study done by *Maes et al.*, some authors reported a significantly weaker correlation between genetics and obesity. Interestingly, other researchers established an even stronger correlation than Stunkard did. The role of genetics in the development of obesity has been studied for decades, however there is no consensus among researchers. There are a lot of conflicting data and reliable estimates are not available. Based on conservative estimates, it is safe to say that the importance of genetic factors in the pathogenesis of obesity should be placed somewhere in the range of 10 to 90%.

PIMA INDIANS - REVISITED

In the previous chapter, we read how obesity became the most devastating epidemic in the history of the Arizona Pima Indians. We saw how these formerly tall and strong Indians became the heaviest ethnic group in the United States. Almost two thirds of the Pima men and three quarters of the women were found to be obese. As a result of the obesity epidemic, one of the highest prevalence rates of type-2 diabetes in the world was found among the Pima, living on the Gila River Indian Reservation in Arizona. In addition to those who live in the United States, there are numerous Pima Indians south of the border in the Mexican states of *Chihuahua* and *Sonora*.

On the Gila River Indian Reservation, 69% of the elderly women were found to be diabetic. The prevalence rate of type-2 diabetes for women among the whole American Pima population was 40%. Here comes the tricky part: only a small fraction of the Mexican Pima suffered from diabetes. The disease was 5.5 times more common in the United States than in Mexico.[38] Obesity showed a similar pattern. The rate of obese Pima men in the U.S. was found to be ten times higher than that in Mexico. As for women, the corresponding obesity ratio was one in three and a half. Furthermore, the Pima in Mexico turned out to be even *healthier than the non-Pima*. How is all that possible?

DNA samples were collected to determine the genetic relationship between the two Pima groups. Based on the analysis of 309 independent markers, American and Mexican Pima Indians are very closely related to each other, although their gene pool is not identical. The Pima living on the south side of the border, also showed a high degree of similarity to other Native-American groups. If Stunkard was right and obesity is in our genes, then how is it possible that two genetically very similar populations like the Pima people of the United States and of Mexico have such a large inequality in their obesity rates? Although the Mexican Pima are prone to obesity, it looks like they have an invisible, life-long protection from obesity, type-2 diabetes and many other diseases. If it is not their genes that keeps them thin, the protective factors must be in their environment. Interestingly, non-Pima Mexicans, whose lifestyle is very similar to the Pima's, have a significantly lower prevalence rate of obesity and diabetes compared to those Mexicans living in Mexico City or in the United States.

The lifestyle of the American and the Mexican Pima Indians differs substantially. The Mexican Pima participate in more physical activities than their American counterparts. On average, the physical activity level of the Pima living in Mexico is 2.5 times higher for men and 7 times higher for women. In addition to different physical activity levels, the diet of the Mexican and the American Pima differs significantly as well. The dietary study of the subjects revealed a major inequality between the two groups. While American Pima consume highly processed foods containing large amounts of refined carbohydrates, the typical diet of the Mexican Pima is rich in fiber and is based on beans, wheat flour tortillas, corn tortillas, and potatoes.

In this section, we compared two groups of people who are closely related to each other, but have a substantially different lifestyle and live in two different environments. One group is thin and healthy, while the other one is obese and suffers from all sorts of diseases. We may ask the question: Is obesity really caused by our genes?

SUMMARY

From the examples seen in this chapter, we can conclude that the role of genes in the development of obesity is far less important than what some experts claim. Although genetics is a crucial part of the equation, genes by themselves do not cause obesity (except for a few extremely rare examples). These rare cases don't make up even one percent of the total number of obese people. What about the other 60% of the population in the industrialized countries who are obese or overweight? There is no doubt that our genes predispose us to obesity. However, it is our lifestyle and the environment that activates those genes and make us obese. The good news is that even if you inherited those nasty obesity genes, they don't have to be expressed. Just keep on reading. Later in this book, I will explain in details what changes in your diet and lifestyle can prevent the expression of your obesity genes and how can you reach your optimal weight and stay lean and healthy for good.

9

FATTENING CARBOHYDRATES

THE PHYSIOLOGY OF TASTE

The foundations of modern nutrition science were laid down as early as 200 years ago. The French polymath, Jean Anthelme Brillat-Savarin's famous work, *The Physiology of Taste* was first published in 1825. The book has been continuously in print for almost two centuries. Brillat-Savarin was born to a family of influential lawyers. He studied law, chemistry and medicine in Dijon and later he became a lawyer. Brillat-Savarin's expertise was not limited to life sciences but he was also a culinary expert. In his book entitled, *The Physiology of Taste,* the author examines the relationship between dietary habits and health; he also dedicated a whole chapter to obesity. We learn from his book that morbidly obese people existed even in the 19th century. He wrote about a friend of his who was about five feet two inches high, but weighed five hundred pounds. However, the most remarkable case Brillat-Savarin ever encountered, was in New York. There was a large man sitting in a chair in the doorway of a café on Broadway. Savarin described his legs as "stout enough to have sustained a church".

The author listed three causes of obesity: First, there are individuals who were born with predisposition to obesity. (That was long before the birth of the science of genetics). Starch is the second cause of obesity. All animals that live on starchy food become fat; man is also subject to this common law. Starchy foods with added sugar are the most fattening ones. The author also noted that: "We never eat sweet things until the appetite is already satisfied, so that we are forced to court the luxury of eating by every refinement of temptation". He pointed out that carbohydrates in beverages are as fattening as those in foods. Beer drinking nations have "huge stomachs". He also mentioned that some Parisian beer drinkers grew big bellies since they could not afford wine. The third cause of obesity is excessive eating and drinking. The human race is the only one that eats without hunger, and drinks without thirst. Animals simply don't do that,

In the history of medicine, Brillat-Savarin was the first one, who studied the underlying causes of obesity, and based his theory on modern scientific principles. Although some of his findings are outdated, he identified the three major risk factors that are associated with obesity: genetics, refined carbohydrates, and binge eating. Unfortunately, his warning about the fattening effect of carbohydrates has been forgotten during the last two centuries.

THE WORLD'S FIRST DIET BOOK

The first diet book was written by *William Banting*, who was an Englishman living in 19th century London. Banting didn't have a formal medical education: by trade, he was a carpenter, undertaker and coffin maker. In his thirties, Banting started to put on some weight. Over the course of the following decades he accumulated a considerable amount of body fat. He wasn't able to find the remedy for his obesity for nearly thirty years. Nothing seemed to work for Banting; he said "the evil still gradually increased". An eminent surgeon and family friend recommended more physical exertion. Following the doctor's advice, Banting started his every morning with vigorous rowing exercise on the nearby Thames river.

Although he gained some muscular strength, regular outdoor activities caused him to develop a very healthy appetite. In the end, rather than losing weight, he became even heavier. The advice Banting was given turned out to be as useless as today's common recipe for weight loss: *"Exercise more and eat less"*. As we have seen in this story, the strategy of increasing the physical activity level fails, not only today, but also failed 150 years ago. As for the second recommendation, ie. "eat less", the calorie reduction approach didn't work for William Banting either. He always felt hungry and tired and ended up eating even more than before. Banting was involved in other forms of physical exercise as well, such as walking and horseback riding, however these activities didn't help him lose weight either. He also tried remedies which today are considered quackery or fad diets like liquor potasse, sea air, or Turkish bath. By 1862, Banting was so obese, that he wasn't able to tie his shoes and had constant joint pains, ear and vision problems.

Then, he came to the attention of a well-known ear surgeon, *William Harvey*, who prescribed a specific diet for Banting. Dr. Harvey spent the early years of his career in Paris, the center of experimental medicine at the time. Banting was told to refrain from bread, butter, milk, sugar, beer, and potatoes, which were the main elements of his diet. On the other hand, meat, fish, fruits and vegetables were allowed. The bread consumption was limited to 1 ounce per meal. As a result of the strict low-carbohydrate diet, Banting managed to lose 46 pounds within one year. He felt much younger and more energetic. The joint pains were gone; he had no more heart burns and he could tie his shoes again. His sight and hearing had greatly improved. Banting was amazed by the results. He authored a booklet entitled: *Letter on Corpulence, Addressed to the Public* which is considered to be the first diet book. Banting approached the editor of *The Lancet* with the manuscript. *The Lancet* was one the most prestigious medical journals back then and still is today. However, the scientific community didn't take the former carpenter seriously. After Banting was turned down by the editor, he self-published the book, which finally became a bestseller and had multiple editions. By the 1870s, the expression "to bant" became synonymous with "to diet".

Although many modern, low-carbohydrate high-fat diets are very similar to the Banting diet, and these schemes have lots of followers even today, there are a few less well-known facts that Banting's fans don't mention. William Banting never reached his normal weight, as some authors claim. From the *obese* category (BMI=33) he went down to be *overweight* (BMI=26). There are many pictures of William Banting available on the internet. If we take a close look at the photo of his whole body, we will notice his strikingly enlarged abdominal fat deposits that remained even after the alleged weight loss. Banting claims that he lost 46 pounds, but we have no information if he also managed to keep the weight off for a longer period of time. This is the Achilles' heel of the diet industry, where every single diet fails in the long run. Last but not least, Banting was a heavy drinker. He writes in his booklet that 4 to 7 glasses of wine were part of his everyday diet. Banting's alcoholism greatly undermines his credibility.

THE FATHER OF MODERN MEDICINE

Sir William Osler was a Canadian physician, often referred to as "the father of modern medicine". In 1892, Dr. Osler published a textbook for practitioners and medical students entitled: *The Principles and Practice of Medicine*. It was translated into several languages and became the most important medical textbook for the next 40 years. For the treatment of obesity, Osler recommended a low-carbohydrate diet, consisting of meat, milk, fruits and vegetables; limiting bread intake to 55 grams (the size of a hamburger bun today) and potato consumption to 100 grams a day. According to Osler's regimen, occasionally a "hunger day" should be also taken. He also recommended that in children's diet starches and fats should be reduced and they are not allowed to eat sweets.

THE 20TH CENTURY

From the early 1800s until the middle of the last century, carbohydrates were generally viewed as the main cause of obesity. Decades before the outbreak of the worldwide obesity epidemic, there were numerous publications dealing with the fattening effects of carbohydrates. Benjamin Spock's *The Common Sense Book of Baby and Child Care* is one of the best-selling books of the twentieth century with over 50 million copies sold. Dr. Spock said in his world-famous book: "Rich desserts can be omitted without risk, and should be, by anyone who is obese and trying to reduce. The amount of plain, starchy foods (cereals, breads, potatoes) taken is what determines, in the case of most people, how much they gain or lose."

In 1963, Dr. Passmore and Dr. Swindells started their article in the *British Journal of Nutrition* with the following statement[39]:

"Every woman knows that carbohydrate is fattening: this is a piece of common knowledge, which few nutritionists would dispute."
Until the 1960s, there was still a consensus among leading scientists about the fattening effect of carbohydrates, as we've seen in Dr. Passmore's article in the *British Journal of Nutrition*.

Heart disease was an uncommon cause of death in the first half of the 20th century. However, things started to change after World War II. With the fast-paced economic growth and industrialization in the Western countries, coronary heart disease became the number one killer of middle-aged men by the 1960s. Since the outbreak of the large heart disease epidemic, researchers were strenuously looking for the answer to the question: What causes heart disease? In the early 1950s, the former marine biologist, *Ancel Keys* came up with a strange theory that coronary heart disease is caused by fat consumption. Those days nobody took him seriously, Keys was often ridiculed for his bold idea. Even Keys himself was a big time skeptic of his own theory. However, at the beginning of the great epidemic of heart disease things started to change rapidly. Governments and health authorities under the pressure from the public needed to find a culprit for the most devastating disease of the 20th century. Dietary fat was an excellent candidate. The fattening effect of carbohydrates was suddenly forgotten and from that point, dietary fat was considered to be one of the major risk factors for cardiovascular disease. We were told by health authorities to reduce our fat intake and consume more carbohydrates instead. Unfortunately, we quickly forgot about the fact that the consumption of refined carbohydrates causes obesity and the whole population was put on a *low-fat, high-carbohydrate diet*.

FORERUNNERS OF THE ATKINS DIET

Today, low-carbohydrate diets are often associated with the name of *Robert Atkins*. However, Dr. Atkins himself didn't really invent anything new, because low-carbohydrate diets have been around since the early 1800s. There was a prominent scientist who prepared the road for the Atkins diet. *Dr. Alfred W. Pennington* was the medical director of duPont. One of his responsibilities was to help company employees lose weight. In a short period of over 100 days he achieved an average 22 pound weight loss per employee by putting the 20 subjects on a strict low-carbohydrate diet. In 1953, Pennington published his article on the treatment of obesity with a calorically unrestricted, low carbohydrate diet.[40] The method described in *Dr. Atkins' Diet Revolution* is based on Pennington's concept.

THE ATKINS DIET

There was a brave man who dared to swim against the tide. His name is Dr. Robert Coleman Atkins, a young cardiologist from New York. Robert Atkins in his thirties started to put on some weight and it made him very frustrated. "I weighed 193 pounds and had three chins. I couldn't get up before 9 a.m. and never saw patients before 10. I decided to go on a diet." - said Dr. Atkins. The young doctor went through the medical literature and settled on the 150 year old *low carbohydrate* method, that was successfully applied by Alfred W. Pennington since the 1940s.

Atkins saw that the low carbohydrate approach does work – at least in the short run. By the end of the first month he managed to lose 20 pounds. Dr. Atkins started prescribing the new diet for his patients as well. The American Telephone and Telegraph Company hired Dr. Atkins as a medical consultant. He treated 65 patients and 64 of them achieved their goal to lose a substantial amount of weight. His first book was published in 1972, entitled *Dr. Atkins' Diet Revolution*. The Atkins diet had a lot of media attention. Atkins suddenly became the most popular diet doctor in the United States. Various editions of the book sold more than 15 million copies, making it one of the best-selling diet books ever written.

Although he was a celebrated national hero, the medical community was not really amazed by Dr. Atkins' revolutionary new ideas. The 1973 *U.S. Senate Select Committee* investigating fad diets said "The Atkins Diet is nonsense". The president of the *American College of Nutrition* said about the diet: "Of all the bizarre diets that have been proposed in the last 50 years, this is the most dangerous to the public if followed for any length of time". The Chair of the *American Medical Association's* Council on Food and Nutrition testified

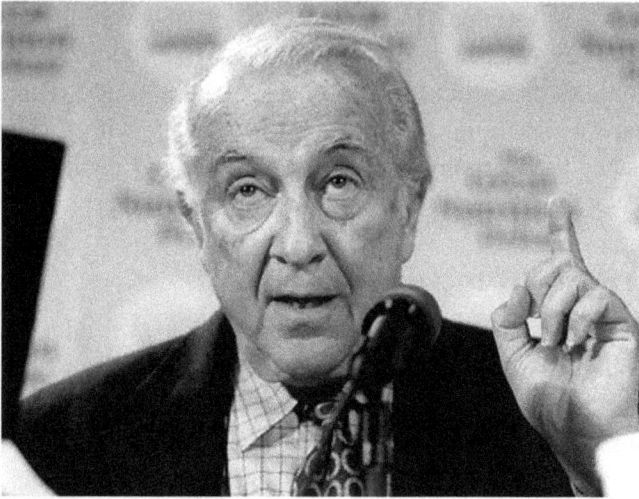

Figure 9.1. Robert Atkins

before the Senate Subcommittee as follows: "It became apparent that the diet as recommended poses a serious threat to health." All the prestigious medical and scientific organizations opposed the Atkins diet, including the *American Medical Association, American Dietetic Association, National Academy of Sciences, American Cancer Society* and the *American Heart Association.* However, Atkins was not discouraged by the criticism and he continued building up his diet empire. Atkins Nutritionals Inc. was selling a whole variety of Atkins approved products. In 2012 the company produced about $311 million in revenue.

The death of Dr. Atkins was even more controversial than his life. In 2003, he fell and suffered a head injury on an icy sidewalk. He was admitted to hospital and underwent surgery to remove a blood clot from his brain. Later, he fell into a coma and died from complications. This is the official version of the story of Dr. Atkins' death. Others claim however, that the famous diet doctor was severely obese and he was diagnosed with heart disease as well.

On February 11, 2004 *The New York Times* published an article entitled *Just What Killed the Diet Doctor, And What Keeps the Issue Alive?*

"The latest twist is the publication in The Wall Street Journal on Tuesday of details from Dr. Atkins's confidential medical report. The report concludes that Dr. Atkins, 72, had a history of heart attack and congestive heart failure and notes that he weighed 258   pounds at death."

Veronica Atkins, Dr. Atkins' widow, had denied that the doctor's heart problems were related to his death. One of his consultants claimed that Dr. Atkins weighed 195 pounds when he was hospitalized. The 63-pound weight gain was caused by fluid retention during the nine days while he was in a coma. For a long period of time, Dr. Atkins suffered from cardiomyopathy, a disease that affects the heart muscle. Very often, the underlying cause of cardiomyopathy remains unknown, so we don't know for sure if Dr. Atkins' own diet can be connected to his death.

However, it is a well-known fact that people who personally knew Dr. Atkins, described the diet doctor as obese. The billionaire *Michael Bloomberg* who was the mayor of New York City at that time, called Atkins "fat" and claimed that he doesn't believe that the accident caused the doctor's death; he called the official version of the story "B.S.". Dr. John McDougall also knew Atkins. He described the diet doctor as "grossly overweight", estimating his weight to be 40 to 60 pounds higher than normal.

Even if we accept Atkins' consultant's statement that the doctor weighed 195 pounds when he was admitted to the hospital, the 6 foot man had a body mass index of 26.4, which is well in the overweight category. At that point, his weight was even two pounds more than at his young age before he invented his infamous diet. There are two possible explanations: either the Atkins diet doesn't work in the long run, or the famous doctor cheated on his own diet. Following the death of Dr. Atkins, the popularity of his controversial diet went into decline. In 2005, Atkins Nutritionals Inc., the former diet empire, filed for bankruptcy. At that time, the company's total loss exceeded $340 million.

Let's take a quick look at the diet itself. It is an undeniable fact that some dieters experience a drastic weight loss during the first week or two after they start the program. However, the results are very questionable, because patients don't lose a large amount of fat. The body stores the excess carbohydrates in the form of glycogen in the skeletal muscles and the liver. Since the Atkins diet is based on carbohydrate restriction, the glycogen reserves of the body are gradually depleted during the initial period of the program. Glycogen tends to retain a large amount of water; most of the experienced weight loss comes from the lower levels of glycogen and water and the reduced amount of food passing through the digestive tract, not from the fat deposits. After the mobilization of the easily accessible substances, the pace of weight loss slows down in most individuals.

Several studies were done to evaluate the long-term effect of the Atkins diet and other low-carbohydrate diets. After analyzing the results of 13 experiments with the participation of 1,222 volunteers, researchers found that in the beginning, low-carbohydrate diets result in a faster weight loss, however subjects tend to regain their original weight after a year.[41]

In the 1972 edition of *Dr. Atkins' Diet Revolution*, the author still claimed that dieters can eat unrestricted amounts of approved food: "You eat as much as you want, as often as you want". The book was never meant to be a scientific work. Certain parts were written by *Ruth West* who was neither scientist nor doctor, but a content writer and marketing executive. In the first edition, authors made several incorrect statements that were erased from the later versions of the book. The "You eat as much as you want, as often as you want" assertion was later changed in the new 2002 edition to "as much as you needed to feel satisfied", which made a huge difference. Atkins' company executives don't like to be reminded of their previous mistakes. *Collette Heimowitz* of Atkins Nutritionals said: "The media and opponents of Atkins often sensationalize and simplify the diet as the all-the-steak-you-can-eat diet. This has never been true."

It is estimated that 20 million people worldwide went on the Atkins diet. Where are the long-term results? For example, we have never heard of people who went on Atkins diet 10 years ago, lost 50 pounds, and have kept the weight off. As a conclusion, the Atkins diet should definitely be put into the fad diet category, especially the original version published in the 1972 edition of the book. Despite the failure of his diet in the long run, Robert Atkins made a valuable contribution to modern nutrition science: in the middle of the cholesterol hysteria, he pointed out the fattening effect of refined carbohydrates, which are closely associated with today's obesity epidemic.

WHY ARE CARBOHYDRATES FATTENING?

The fattening effect of carbohydrates has been a well-known fact for 200 years, as we saw it in the previous examples of Brillat-Savarin, William Banting, William Osler, Alfred W. Pennington, Robert Atkins and others. Although we knew for a long time that carbohydrates caused obesity, we didn't really know why. Carbohydrates are very energy-dense nutrients; each gram of carbohydrate contains over 4 kilocalories. A plausible explanation is that the calories contained in carbohydrates make us obese. It is true to a certain degree, but we will discuss in the next chapter that the *calories in-calories out* model by itself cannot explain the causes of obesity. You may ask the question: in addition to the carbohydrates' high energy content, are there any other reasons as well?

Everybody has heard about insulin; most of us associate it with diabetes. Insulin was first isolated by the Canadian physician *Frederick Banting,* who was also the first one to treat diabetic patients with insulin. In healthy individuals, insulin is produced by the beta cells of the pancreas. Type-1 diabetes is a disease characterized by low or no insulin production, which is caused by the destruction of the pancreatic beta cells. In patients with type-2 diabetes, the pancreas produces insulin, but the body does not respond normally to the hormone. This condition is known as *insulin resistance.* Obesity and insulin resistance are closely related to each other. Most people who suffer from type-2 diabetes are also obese. Conversely, many obese individuals have an impaired insulin sensitivity, and are at a higher risk to develop diabetes over time.

Insulin is widely known for its blood sugar-lowering effect. That's why diabetic patients use insulin. It is a less well-known fact that insulin is an anabolic hormone. Besides controlling blood sugar levels, insulin has other functions as well; it promotes fat storage and the conversion of excess sugar into glycogen. Insulin also increases protein synthesis and cell growth. Because of its anabolic properties, insulin is the main driving force behind obesity.

Shortly after food consumption, the pancreas releases insulin into the bloodstream. Originally, it was thought that only carbohydrates could trigger a post-meal insulin response, and scientists did not pay too much attention to the difference between various types of carbohydrates. It turned out however, that certain amino acids from protein rich foods can also increase insulin secretion[4]. As for carbohydrates, it makes a huge difference what type of carbohydrates we consume. Highly refined ones, especially sugar and starch cause a sudden spike in both blood sugar and insulin levels. However, following the initial insulin rush, within a short period of time, blood sugar drops faster than normal and we feel hungry again. That's the reason why it's so hard to satisfy our hunger with foods that contain high amounts of refined carbohydrates such as sugar and starch. *Part IV* of this book will discuss in detail how to distinguish between "good" and "bad" carbohydrates.

10

CALORIES IN, CALORIES OUT

WHAT IS A CALORIE?

Calorie is one of the most frequently used words these days. Not a single day passes without coming across the ominous word on food labels, commercials, newspaper articles, the internet and other media as well. What is exactly a calorie? A calorie is a unit of energy. One calorie is the amount of energy needed to raise the temperature of 1 gram of water by 1 degree Celsius. One *kilocalorie* equals one thousand calories. Causing lots of confusion, the popular media uses the units *calorie* and *kilocalorie* interchangeably. Although it's not entirely correct, in this context the term *calorie* means *kilocalorie* or *nutritional calorie*.

A calorimeter is a device that measures the energy content of various food items (see Figure 10.1). The first calorimeter was built by the French chemist *Antoine Lavoisier* in the late 1700s.

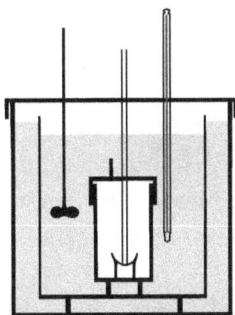

Figure 10.1. Bomb calorimeter
The device consists of a container full of water, and a combustion chamber where the food sample is burned in the presence of oxygen. The energy content of the food is calculated from the water's temperature rise in the tank.

WE WERE TOLD THAT "A CALORIE IS A CALORIE"

The energy content of various food items was first measured by German scientist *Max Rubner* at the end of the 19th century. Using a calorimeter, Rubner calculated the caloric value of food from carbohydrates, fats and proteins. He found that the available energy absorbed through digestion is always less than the energy gained by experimentally burning different foods, because a portion of the nutrients passes through the human body undigested. An adjustment was applied for each type of food for its indigestible portion. Rubner's *isodynamic law* says that for energy purposes different foods may replace one another in accordance with their caloric values. Today's notion that *a calorie is a calorie* is based on Rubner's isodynamic law. In addition to the isodynamic law, Rubner also described the *law of surface area:* the energy expenditure of the animals is proportional to their body's surface area.

Following Max Rubner, *Wilbur Olin Atwater* in the United States had also calculated the nutritional value of macronutrients by using similar calorimetric methods. He determined the energy content of carbohydrates and proteins to be 4.1 kcal per gram and of fats 9.3 kcal per gram. Atwater's method was used for decades thereafter.

Food labeling has been mandatory in many countries since the end of the last century. Calories however are no longer determined directly by burning the foods in a calorimeter. Total energy content is calculated by adding up the calories from each energy-containing nutrient: protein, carbohydrate and fat.

WHEN TWO PLUS TWO EQUALS FIVE

Although several hypotheses are used to explain what causes obesity, the *calories in - calories out* model is the predominant view among researchers and healthcare professionals. The *World Health Organization* (WHO) is no exception either. As per the WHO website: "The fundamental cause of obesity and overweight is an energy imbalance between calories consumed and calories expended."

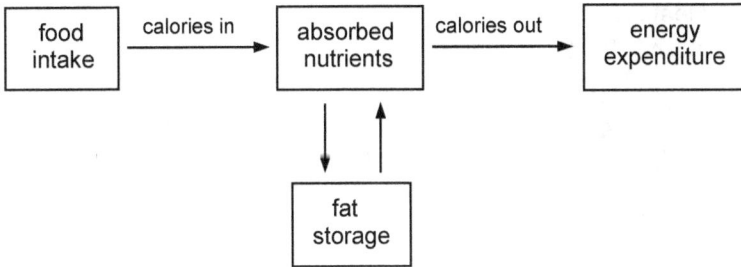

Figure 10.2. The calories in - calories out model

Nutrients are absorbed from the ingested food (calories in). The energy from the food is used for maintaining vital body functions, growth, physical activity etc. (calories out). The excess energy will be stored in the form of body fat (positive energy balance). If energy expenditure exceeds energy intake, the energy shortage will be supplied from the stored fat (negative energy balance, see Figure 10.2). In other words, if we eat too much and exercise too little, sooner or later we will be fat. Conversely, to lose weight, the only thing we need to do is slightly reduce our meal portion sizes or do some exercising once in a while. Now, our energy balance is negative and we've immediately started to lose weight. It is just a question of time, and we will go back to our high school weight.

Let me tell you an exaggerated example. Let's say you cut back your food intake by a 100 calories a day. Not a big deal; you won't even notice a 100 calories. Even one single chocolate chip cookie has more than a 100 calories. We have all heard the saying, "Little things add up". With minimal effort, your annual energy intake is reduced by 36,500 calories and you will have managed to lose 10 pounds during the first year alone! This is just the beginning. Within a few years, you will be even slimmer than you were back in high school. In a couple of decades, your body will weigh virtually zero. ☺

Proponents of the *calories in - calories out* model often refer to the *first law of thermodynamics*: energy can be neither created nor destroyed. Of course, the *first law of thermodynamics* is true, being one of nature's most fundamental laws, however it is completely

Heat loss

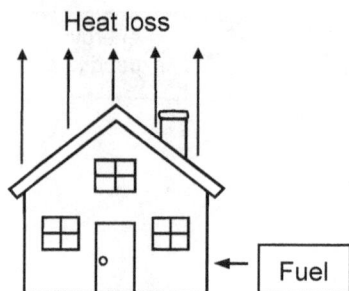

Figure 10.3. The calories in - calories out model. With a constant indoor temperature, the energy supplied by the fuel (calories in) equals the total heat loss (calories out).

irrelevant to obesity. For example, you can apply the *first law of thermodynamics* when analyzing the energy balance of your house (see Figure 10.3), but the law of energy conservation by itself can't explain the causes of obesity. Living organisms are way more complicated than a building with walls, roof, windows, doors and a furnace. Every single process in our body is precisely regulated by hormones and other chemical signaling molecules. Weight gain and weight loss is no exception. In addition to hormones, there are other factors as well that regulate body weight. The problem with the *calories in - calories out* model is that it grossly oversimplifies human metabolism.

"A calorie is a calorie" – says mainstream nutrition science. Let's take a closer look at what is wrong with the most common nutrition myth ever. What will happen if a 100 calories of sugar or a 100 calories of raw cabbage are burned in a lab environment? As expected, both foods will produce the same amount of heat. You've already heard the saying "A calorie is a calorie". It is 100% correct in the food scientists' bomb calorimeters for sure. These two foods however have very different effects on the human metabolism. Sugar is a very energy-dense food; 100 calories are packed into a small amount of 25 grams only, which is the equivalent of two tablespoons. Shortly after ingestion, the sugar will cause a sudden spike in the blood glucose level, followed by an insulin rush. Insulin is an anabolic hormone and it is the main driving force behind obesity. Insulin works hard to put every possible food item into storage for later use. It acts like a squirrel or hamster. After the initial blood sugar peak however, the blood glucose level will drop faster than normal and you will be even hungrier than before. As a result you will end up eating more food.

Cabbage on the other hand, is not an energy-dense food. In order to consume 100 calories you have to eat 400 grams of it, which is half of a medium sized cabbage. Besides calories, cabbage also contains fiber and a lot of water. By slowing down nutrient absorption, fibers prevent enormous fluctuations in blood sugar levels. Since there are no sharp blood sugar spikes, insulin levels also remain stable. Fewer nutrients will be stored as fat. As we've seen in the previous example, it makes a huge difference what source the same amount of energy comes from. Fats, proteins and carbohydrates are all metabolized differently; even nutrients within the carbohydrate group such as glucose, fructose, sucrose or starch have very different effects on our metabolism.

ERRONEOUS ASSUMPTIONS

The *calories in - calories out* model assumes that our caloric intake has no effect on our caloric expenditure. Many of those who are on a low-calorie diet feel cold all the time, because the human body reacts to severe caloric restrictions by slowing down the basal metabolic rate and switching to energy-saving mode. On the other hand, after a generous sized holiday meal you may feel excessively hot, because your body produces more heat from the excess calories. In other words, a higher caloric intake results in a higher caloric expenditure and a lower caloric intake causes a lower caloric expenditure. The association between energy input and output has been studied in several experiments.

From 1944 to 1945, Dr. Ancel Keys and his colleagues conducted a study on human starvation at the University of Minnesota. The trial later became famous as the *Minnesota Starvation Experiment.* During World War II, 36 conscientious objectors – who refused to perform military service – participated in the study. The study's main goal was observing the physical and psychological effects of semistarvation in order to help the rehabilitation of civilians who suffered from undernutrition during the war. In the first three months, the participants received a standard diet of 3,200 calories a day.[42] This was followed by a six-month semistarvation period with an average of 1,570 calories per day. The starvation diet consisted of similar foods to those that were available in wartime Europe; mostly potatoes, turnips, dark bread and macaroni, serving two meals a day. Between the meals, the men were allowed to consume unlimited water, black coffee and chewing gum.

The subjects maintained an active lifestyle, working their regular jobs and in addition to that, they were also required to walk 22 miles a week. Researchers estimated that the participants were expected to burn 3,009 calories a day. However, the energy expenditure of the subjects turned out to be much lower than that. Keys measured a 21-percent reduction in the men's strength and their heart rate slowed down dramatically from 55 to 35 beats per minute. Their metabolic rates went down noticeably and they felt cold all the time. By the end of the experiment, the participants lost 37 pounds on average. The actual weight loss was found to be only half of the amount calculated by the *calories in-calories out* model.

In the United States, with the participation of 48,835 postmenopausal women aged 50 to 79 years, a study was done known as the *Women's Health Initiative Dietary Modification Trial.* One group of the participants was assigned to follow a low-fat diet with caloric restriction, while the other group continued their usual diets with their daily energy intake reduced by 225 kcal. After eight years, researchers compared the occurrence rates of cancer, heart disease, stroke and obesity between the two groups. The results have disproved the accuracy of the *calories in-calories out model.* At the end of the experiment, the weight of the participants was compared to their baseline weight. Those women whose caloric intake was reduced by 225 kcal a day, on average weighed the same eight years later as at the beginning of the experiment. Those who were obese (BMI>30) lost some weight, the overweight subjects (BMI 25-30) kept the weight on, and after 8 years, the normal-weight women got even heavier, despite the caloric restrictions.[43]

SUMMARY

Today's mainstream medicine considers obesity as a result of a caloric imbalance between energy intake and energy expenditure. Therefore, the conventional treatment of obesity is also based on the same idea: in order to lose weight, we should *eat less and exercise more* Over the past few decades however, the *calories in-calories out* model turned out to be wrong. Although, each year millions of dieters torture themselves by fanatically reducing their food intake and increasing their energy expenditure, none of these methods work in the long run. Following an initial weight loss, dieters tend to gain the original weight back within a short period of time. Although the *first law of thermodynamics* itself is correct, the *calories in - calories out* model can not fully explain the cause of obesity.

11

THE BIG FAT MYTH

IS FAT REALLY FATTENING?

At the beginning of the 20th century, coronary heart disease was an uncommon cause of death. Doctors hardly encountered the disease; medical students considered themselves very lucky if they were able to study a single case at all. After World War II however, the prevalence of coronary heart disease had significantly increased along with fast-paced economic growth. By the 1960s, heart disease became the most common cause of death in the United States.

Former marine biologist, Ancel Keys observed that the coronary heart disease mortality rates in Italy are just a fraction of the mortality rates in the United States. Keys also noticed that Italians eat only half as much fat as Americans do. He hypothesized that heart disease is caused by high fat consumption. Keys cherry-picked six countries and created his famous graph drawn with a nearly perfect trend line. In 1953, Keys published his theory in the *Journal of the Mount Sinai Hospital*: the *diet-heart hypothesis* was born. Those days, back in the 1950s, nobody really took him seriously, and Keys was often ridiculed for his bold idea. Even Keys himself was a big time skeptic of his own theory. However, at the beginning of the great epidemic of heart disease, things started to change rapidly. Governments and health authorities under pressure from the public, needed to find a culprit for the most devastating disease of the 20th century. Dietary fat was an excellent candidate. The fattening effect of carbohydrates was suddenly forgotten and from that point on, dietary fat was considered to be the one of the major risk factors for cardiovascular disease. Keys' diet-heart idea had an enormous impact on medical research, health care, and the food industry. The foundations of a multi-billion dollar healthcare, pharmaceutical, food and fitness business were laid on this very fragile *diet-heart hypothesis.* Since then, two generations have already grown up, having been taught that heart disease and fat consumption are closely related. Everybody considers the harmful effects of dietary fat as an unquestionable scientific fact, much like gravity or Pythagoras' Theorem, rather than just a hypothesis, although the proof is scarce. Because coronary artery disease was blamed on dietary fat, it was also assumed that fat consumption causes obesity, although there was no scientific evidence for this claim.

WE WERE GIVEN BAD ADVICE

The United States Senate's *Select Committee on Nutrition and Human Needs* published a pamphlet back in 1977, entitled *Dietary Goals for the United States.* This publication was a turning point in the history of nutrition science: it was the first time ever that the government told people to reduce their fat consumption. According to the pamphlet, dietary goal number one was to "Increase carbohydrate consumption to account for 55 to 60 percent of the energy (caloric) intake." Goal number two was to reduce overall fat consumption from approximately 40 to 30 percent of total energy intake. People listened to their health authorities. The majority of Americans made gigantic efforts to reduce their fat intake and increase their carbohydrate consumption. The food industry lined up quickly with the new ideology, and they flooded the market with their low-fat but highly-processed products. New items emerged on the shelves of grocery stores such as lean meat, low-fat milk and dairy. Food companies don't lack creativity; from time to time they came up with such absurd products like low-fat margarine or low-fat mayonnaise. Food manufacturers know that without fat, their products would taste no better than sawdust. To make their food still palatable, they loaded the new "healthy" foods with lots of sugar. Not to mention the extra salt, artificial flavors, MSG, coloring and other additives. The irony of the low-fat craze is that the overall fat consumption in the United States wasn't reduced at all; it has been steadily increasing since 1960. Although lean meat products, low-fat milk and dairy are more popular than ever, at the end of the day, we eat more fat from French fries, donuts, chocolate and other processed food items. The end result is devastating. Low-fat products are even more fattening than the regular ones. Remarkably, the introduction of the *Dietary Goals for the United States* coincided with the beginning of the largest obesity epidemic in human history. We were given bad advice again.

FATS VS. CARBOHYDRATES

Fats are very energy-dense nutrients and they contain more than twice as much energy as carbohydrates (9.3 vs. 4.1 kcal per gram). In addition to the different energy content, the metabolism of the two groups is substantially different as well. Digested carbohydrates are broken down into simple sugar units resulting in elevated blood glucose levels followed by an insulin rush. Insulin is an anabolic hormone that works hard to put the excess calories into fat storage. Dietary fats, on the other hand, have no significant effect on blood insulin level. The energy-dense fats are less fattening than carbohydrates per energy content. For example, if we compare 100 calories of fats to 100 calories of carbohydrates, fats will show a less obesogenic (fattening) effect because they don't provoke insulin secretion. Not all calories are created equal.

A study was done in Canada, at the University of Toronto to evaluate how fats affect carbohydrate digestion.[44] It was hypothesized that dietary fats and proteins slow down the absorption of carbohydrates. Subjects consumed sugar with various amounts of protein and fat. After each meal, blood samples were taken and researchers measured blood sugar levels. It was found that fats by themselves have just a minimal blood glucose lowering effect taken with a carbohydrate meal. However, if both dietary fats and proteins are added to carbohydrate rich foods, the two nutrients together can slow down the absorption of carbohydrates by up to 21%. Lower blood glucose levels trigger a less intense insulin response. As discussed earlier, insulin is the main driving force behind obesity.

In the previous chapter, we mentioned the *Women's Health Initiative Dietary Modification Trial.* One group of the participants was assigned to follow a low-fat diet with a caloric reduction of 343 kcal / day, while the other group continued their usual diets with their daily energy intake reduced by 225 kcal. At the end of year one, the first group with a low-fat diet and less energy intake lost 2.2 kg on average. By the ninth year, however the difference between the two groups gradually disappeared and the *low-fat and less energy intake* group weighed only 0.6 kg less then the control.[43]

Some experts believe that high dietary fat intake per se leads to obesity, although there is no scientific evidence that could support this hypothesis. The proponents of this theory argue that the prevalence rate of obesity in wealthy countries with high fat intake is significantly higher than in the developing countries with low fat consumption. However, this comparison is very misleading, because there are numerous other confounding factors as well, such as the availability of food, physical activity levels, different lifestyles and the diversity of the countries.

W. C. Willett from *Harvard School of Public Health* combined the results of several clinical trials to determine if low-fat diets have any positive effect on weight loss.[45] Willett found no relationship between fat consumption and obesity. In the conclusion of his study, Willett says:

"Diets high in fat do not account for the high prevalence of excess body fat in Western countries; reductions in the percentage of energy from fat will have no important benefits and could further exacerbate this problem. The emphasis on total fat reduction has been a serious distraction in efforts to control obesity and improve health in general."

We can conclude that fats are not fattening per se. Although they are energy-dense nutrients, fats together with proteins slow down carbohydrate absorption rates, resulting in a less-intense insulin response following a carbohydrate meal. Therefore, switching to a low-fat diet is harmful rather than beneficial.

12

HORMONAL OBESITY

INSULIN IS THE MAIN CULPRIT

Although the *calories in - calories out* theory has been the dominant view to explain obesity for at least half a century, the *carbohydrate-insulin model* has been in existence as an alternative hypothesis for decades as well. In spite of the fact that the fattening effect of carbohydrates has been known for 200 years and insulin was discovered in the early 1900s, nobody really connected insulin with obesity until the second half of the last century. In 1972, among the first ones, Robert Atkins emphasized in his *Diet Revolution* book that excessive carbohydrate intake results in high insulin levels, which leads to obesity. The Atkins diet is based on the same principles that are known today as the *carbohydrate-insulin model.*

Insulin and *glucagon* are the two hormones that directly control blood sugar levels. Both are produced by the pancreas, a slender glandular organ located behind the stomach. The presence of food in the intestines triggers insulin production. The primary function of insulin is to facilitate the uptake of glucose into the cells of the body. Insulin is an anabolic hormone. Besides controlling blood sugar levels, it has other functions as well, such as promoting fat storage and the conversion of excess sugar into glycogen. On the other hand, *glucagon* has just the opposite effect. As a result of low blood glucose levels, the pancreas releases glucagon. The main role of glucagon is to increase blood sugar levels. It is a catabolic hormone, stimulating the mobilization of the stored energy from body fat and glycogen.

The *carbohydrate-insulin model* proposes that foods rich in carbohydrates, especially in sugar and starch, produce hyperinsulinemia, a condition with higher than normal levels of insulin in the blood.

Elevated insulin levels promote the deposit of calories in fat cells instead of utilizing the energy in lean tissues, ultimately leading to obesity (see Figure 12.1).

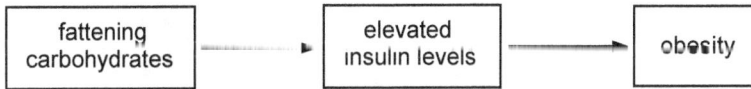

Figure 12.1. The carbohydrate-insulin model

THE VICIOUS CYCLE

The basic principle of the *carbohydrate-insulin model* is correct. Refined carbohydrates do cause obesity and their fattening effect has been known for two centuries. However the *carbohydrate-insulin theory* is incomplete. It lacks one of the crucial elements of obesity: the time factor. People who have been obese for most of their lives may find it extremely difficult to lose weight. In contrast, those who have become obese just recently, can get rid of their excess pounds with considerably less effort. How is it possible?

The previously discussed models of obesity, including the *carbohydrate-insulin theory,* don't take the time factor into consideration. From their point of view it makes no difference if you have been obese for just one year or fifty years. This assumption is not correct, however. The length of obesity has a serious impact on the body's insulin sensitivity. Over time, obese people tend to develop insulin resistance. The longer the duration of obesity, the worse insulin resistance gets. The main function of insulin is assisting cells to uptake circulating glucose from the bloodstream. As obesity progresses, the cells of the human body gradually become desensitized to insulin's effect. With an impaired insulin sensitivity, cells can't absorb as much sugar as they normally would. As a consequence, unabsorbed glucose molecules pile up in the blood. In contrast, body cells go into starvation mode due to the low glucose levels inside the cells. Rising blood glucose levels provoke more insulin secretion. Higher blood insulin levels further exacerbate insulin resistance, forming a vicious cycle (see Figure 12.2).

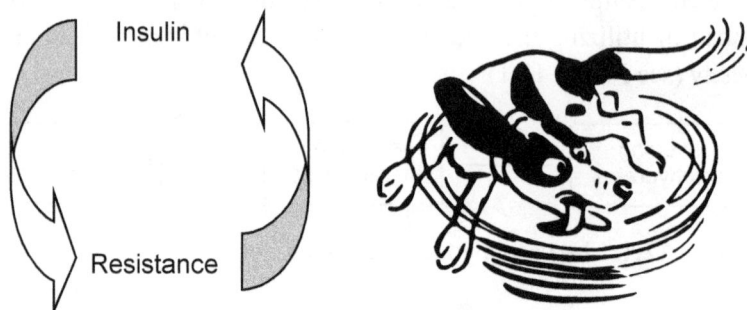

Figure 12.2. The vicious cycle of insulin resistance

By adding the concept of *insulin resistance* to our *carbohydrate-insulin theory* we took one more step toward solving the mystery of obesity. However, our model is not complete yet; there are many other factors that need to be incorporated as well.

CORTISOL

The adrenal hormone *cortisol* plays the second most important role after insulin in the development of obesity. In response to long-term stress exposure, adrenal glands secrete cortisol. The fattening effects of cortisol have been well known for a century. A typical example is *Cushing syndrome* which was named after Harvey Cushing, who first described the disorder. The disease is caused by excessive cortisol production. Rapid weight gain, especially in the trunk and face region is one of the most apparent symptoms of Cushing syndrome. In contrast, those who suffer from Addison's disease, have insufficient cortisol production and they are very thin. There is a clear causal relationship between high cortisol levels and obesity, especially abdominal obesity. Long-term stress is one of the key contributing factors in the development of not only obesity but also diabetes, cardiovascular disease and numerous other serious health conditions. Directly reducing our stress level is very difficult, however getting an adequate amount of sleep may significantly lower our stress and cortisol levels.

Cappuccio et al. studied the relationship between the duration of sleep and obesity.[46] Researchers combined data from numerous clinical trials with over 600,000 participants. The studies showed a strong negative correlation between sleep duration and obesity. On average, one hour of sleep reduction is associated with a 0.35 kg/m² increase in body mass index. In addition to causing elevated cortisol levels, sleep deprivation also interferes with two other hormones: leptin and ghrelin, ultimately leading to increased appetite.

LEPTIN

In addition to insulin and cortisol, the protein hormone *leptin* plays a very important role in the regulation of our body weight as well. Leptin is secreted by fat cells in response to food consumption. Although leptin's primary function is suppressing appetite, it also regulates energy expenditure, coordinates the immune system and affects growth. Since leptin is produced by fat cells, it sounds reasonable that the level of circulating leptin is higher in obese individuals compared to lean people. Following the pattern of insulin resistance, obese people also tend to develop leptin resistance as a result of elevated leptin levels.

Over the course of the last few decades, several experiments were made to treat obesity with exogenous leptin. Although impressive results were achieved in the treatment of patients with leptin gene mutation (those individuals with little or no leptin production), leptin replacement therapy is not suitable to treat common obesity.[47] In the case of obese patients who have already developed leptin resistance, the addition of exogenous leptin doesn't substantially increase its action. As for the treatment of leptin resistant individuals, future research should focus on improving the body's leptin responsiveness instead.

GHRELIN

Ghrelin earned its bad reputation as the "hunger hormone". In a fasting state, ghrelin is produced by the *mucosa*, the inner lining of the stomach. Ghrelin's main function is to increase appetite. When the stomach is stretched, secretion stops. Besides the regulation of appetite, the hormone also controls glucose metabolism and fat storage. Ghrelin is a very controversial hormone and its exact mechanism of action is not well understood. An interesting fact is that obese individuals have a lower level of circulating ghrelin than normal-weight people. Conversely, after weight loss the ghrelin levels return to normal.[48]

OTHER HORMONES

After the major players, let's see the sidekicks. Individually, they don't have a major influence on obesity, but their combined effect may have a significant impact on body weight.

Thyroid hormones have a complex relationship with other hormones. Hypothyroidism (low levels of thyroid hormones) lowers your metabolic rate and ultimately leads to obesity. In contrast, hyperthyroidism (abnormally high levels of thyroid hormones) increases your metabolic rate and causes weight loss.

Adrenalin and noradrenalin help burn calories by increasing heart rate, blood pressure, and other physiological processes associated with energy expenditure. Obesity and overweight are correlated with low levels of testosterone in men. Growth hormone stimulates the breakdown of body fat and the use of stored glycogen in the liver. The role of estrogens in the development of obesity is controversial. In women, estrogens stimulate the formation of fat deposits in certain areas of the body. On the other hand, in post-menopausal women low estrogen levels promote abdominal fat accumulation.

In this chapter, we saw that obesity is not just about nutrients and calories; our body weight is precisely regulated by a whole array of hormones. The model of obesity however is not complete yet. In the following chapters, we will read about other factors as well that play a very important role within the development of obesity.

13

WHAT TO EAT VS. WHEN TO EAT

THE ESSENCE OF TIME

In the previous chapters, we discussed the role of genetics in the development of obesity, we saw how nutrients and calories influence weight gain, and went through the hormonal theory of obesity. We concluded that among all hormones, insulin is the chief regulator of our body weight. Following a carbohydrate meal, digested starch and compound sugars are broken down into simple sugar units and are taken up by the circulation. The absorbed carbohydrates increase blood glucose levels. Rising blood sugar levels trigger an insulin response. Besides regulating blood glucose, insulin has a secondary function as well: it diverts nutrients into the fat deposits. From a nutritional point of view, insulin can be viewed as the main driving force behind obesity.

We haven't mentioned yet the importance of timing. The fattening effect of foods depends not only on the food itself, but is also significantly influenced by the time of the day the meal is consumed. In other words, the question of *when to eat* is almost as important as *what to eat*. There is an old proverb that says, "Eat breakfast like a king, lunch like a prince, and dinner like a pauper". Although the adage is not entirely correct, there is a lot wisdom in it. This saying points out the importance of timing. The bulk of our caloric intake should be allocated between the morning hours and noon. Let's take a closer look why. For example, if you eat two identical meals, one served in the morning and one in the evening, they don't have the same fattening effect. As many people might suspect, the same food consumed in the evening causes more weight gain than if it is eaten in the morning.

Physiological processes in our bodies show a daily pattern, called the *circadian rhythm*. For example, *melatonin*, the hormone causing sleepiness is produced in largest quantities during the evening hours and at night. Just like the other hormones, insulin secretion shows its own similar daily pattern as well.

An experiment was conducted with the participation of twenty healthy volunteers to study how the timing of each meal affects blood glucose levels and insulin production.[49] Subjects were served three identical meals per day. Researchers found that the group served the same meal in the evening shows a 75% increase in blood sugar levels, over and above the increase among the group that is served the same meal in the morning. In addition to that, the body's insulin sensitivity is significantly higher in the morning hours than later during the day.

We can conclude that the same meal has a significantly less fattening effect in the morning than in the evening. The phenomenon can be partially explained by higher insulin sensitivity in the early hours and by the changing daily patterns of the secretion of other hormones as well. Another possible explanation, is that during the day we are physically more active and expend more calories than in the evening hours.

INTERMITTENT FASTING

The term *intermittent fasting* may sound familiar for many of us. From time to time, we come across this very popular but controversial topic in social media, videos, newspaper articles and on television. Unfortunately, mainstream science hasn't really discovered the great potential of this simple, yet extremely efficient tool that is not only more powerful than any other weight-loss methods, but it is also absolutely free! Fasting is not only free, but you will even save money, because you don't need to spend it on weight-loss programs, food supplements or medication. Curious readers may ask the question: if fasting is so good for us, why is it not recommended to us by our doctors, dieticians, pharmacists and health advisors? The answer is very simple. Since fasting is free, nobody really makes money if you fast. Our profit-oriented Western medicine, instead of preventing the underlying causes of diseases, uses expensive drugs to suppress the symptoms, without curing the disease itself.

Intermittent fasting is the most important element of both weight-loss and weight maintenance regimens. There are many different versions of intermittent fasting. The common feature of all protocols is refraining from food and caloric beverages for an extended period of time. The typical length of the fasting interval is 24 hours, but it can also be shorter or longer. A fasting day is either followed by a regular eating day or another fasting day. If you have two or more fasting days in a row, after each fasting day, you will have a meal. It's up to you to see how many fasting days you can commit to yourself. It can be as little as just one day a week or as many as seven days a week. The higher the level of commitment, the faster the results.

Alternate day fasting involves an alternating dietary pattern: every fasting day is followed by a feeding day. On fasting days, some authors allow a limited amount of food intake;[50] however strict protocols prohibit food consumption on fasting days. In my opinion, on fasting days, we should completely refrain from food and caloric beverages. If we just keep on eating on fasting days, we can not really call it fasting, but rather a calorie-restricted diet, which does not work in the long run.

Let's see the scientific explanations of how intermittent fasting works. From the *calories in-calories out* perspective, weight loss is a result of a negative energy balance. While fasting, since there is virtually zero caloric intake, the body starts utilizing the energy stored in the form of glycogen and body fat. Although there are certain elements of truth in this explanation, the caloric model grossly oversimplifies the problem. In the *Hormonal Obesity* chapter, we saw that besides nutrients and calories, our body weight is precisely regulated by a whole array of hormones as well.

Insulin is the chief regulator of our energy metabolism. The hormone's main function is helping the body's cells to absorb the glucose from the bloodstream. Every skeletal muscle and fat cell of our body has insulin receptors. Let's say they are the keyholes. Insulin is the key. It opens up the transport channels which let glucose inside the cells. This is the way that glucose metabolism works in *healthy* individuals.

However, as obesity progresses, the cells of the human body gradually become desensitized to insulin's effect. With an impaired insulin sensitivity, cells can't absorb as much sugar as they would normally. As a consequence, unabsorbed glucose molecules pile up in the blood. In contrast, body cells go into starvation mode due to the low glucose levels inside the cells. Rising blood glucose levels provoke more insulin secretion. Higher blood insulin levels further exacerbate insulin resistance, forming a vicious cycle (see Figure 12.2).

Let's see how can you break the vicious cycle of insulin resistance. While fasting, despite zero caloric intake, the body's homeostasis still needs to be maintained. In order to provide the cells with fuel, the body will be looking for alternative fuels. After using up exogenous sugar, the glycogen reserves of the liver and muscles will be gradually converted into sugar. This new energy source keeps you moving for another half a day or so. Once glycogen stores are depleted, then comes the fat. Fat is quite an energy-dense substance. Theoretically, if you are a normal-weight person who stopped eating entirely, your body fat would keep you alive for another month or two; it greatly depends on the individual's fat reserves. According to the *Guinness Book of World Records*, the longest recorded fast lasted for 382 days. Although most healthy people would survive even for weeks without food, in your regimen, the length of a typical fasting period doesn't need to be more than 24-36 hours. To achieve a fast, but sustainable weight-loss effect, 24-hour fasting days are long enough in the case of most individuals. In order to avoid the loss of lean body mass, the duration of fast should not be longer than 48 hours. In contrast to traditional calorie-restricted diets, which turned out to be a complete failure in the long run, intermittent fasting offers numerous health benefits:

1. Since your energy intake equals zero, your body has no other choice than burning your own fat. This rarely happens with calorie-restricted diets.

2. Continuously low insulin levels will help you restore your body's insulin sensitivity. Since the body gradually gets more and more sensitive to insulin's effects, the pancreas has to secrete less and less insulin. The vicious cycle of insulin resistance will be turned back little by little, day by day. For the first time in your life, you will treat the underlying cause of obesity, not just the symptoms.

3. Reset your inner "body weight thermostat". Many dieters, even those who are brave enough to go through a hardcore diet program, and successfully lost a considerable amount of weight, will run into the same problem. Within a few months or in a year, the pounds they lost will gradually come back, and they will end up weighing the same or probably even more than before. It seems like there is an invisible mechanism which controls body weight. Our body desperately defends our preset weight. The weight regulator keeps the same body weight in the long run, just like the thermostat regulates the temperature of your house. Besides bariatric surgery, fasting is the most efficient way to re-program your inner "body weight thermostat".

4. Detoxify your body. People spend a *healthy* amount of money on vitamins, food supplements, and detoxifying cures just to get rid of the "hazardous waste" inside. Fasting works, guaranteed.

THE EATING WINDOW

It's an amazing fact that the introduction of the new dietary guidelines in 1977, called *Dietary Goals for the United States* coincided with the beginning of the greatest obesity epidemic ever. For the first time in history, the government told the citizens to cut back their fat intake and consume more carbohydrates. We were also encouraged to snack between our three regular meals. Unfortunately, people took the bad advice: reduced their fat intake, increased carbohydrate consumption, and developed a new habit of constant grazing. As a result, the population grew heavier and heavier each year. To illustrate the absurdity of what health authorities called healthy a few decades ago, here are some excerpts from the 1991 pamphlet *The American Heart Association* (AHA) *Diet: An Eating Plan for Healthy Americans.* From the group *Breads, Cereals, Pasta and Starchy Vegetables, AHA* recommended six or more servings a day. The list of "healthy" foods included: white bread, hard candy, gum drops, sugar, syrup, honey, jam, jelly, marmalade, fruit punches and carbonated soft drinks. They even recommended up to 12 ounces (0.36 liters) of beer (!) in the list of healthy foods.

Until the 1970s, most people had only three meals a day, typically prepared at home. Over the course of the past four decades however, homemade meals have been gradually replaced with fast food. The quality of the food we eat has changed substantially as well as the frequency of our food intake. Under the pressure of health "experts" and television commercials, three additional meals were squeezed between our regular breakfast, lunch and dinner. By taking advantage of the new dietary guidelines, over the last couple of decades, a very lucrative snack food industry was built on the new concept of constant grazing. By the early 2000s, over 60% of Americans ate a snack at least 3 times a day. By 2006, in the United States, the energy intake from snacking totaled 679 kcalories a day.[51] You may ask the question: why is snacking a bad habit? There are several reasons. First, from the traditional view point, snackers consume a lot of extra calories that they normally wouldn't. In order to avoid the intake of these extra calories, the sizes of our regular meals have to be cut down, which will lead to a state of constant hunger. In addition to that, pretty much all of the snack food items fall into the junk food category: they tend to contain high amounts of refined carbohydrates, salt, additives and trans fat. This is not all. The worst part is still to come: it's insulin, the CEO of your energy management company.

Figure 13.1 shows the simplified daily insulin secretion curve for a traditional, *3 meals per day* dietary pattern. Shortly after the ingestion of each meal, nutrient absorption is followed by a sharp increase in both blood glucose and insulin levels. Between meals and during the nighttime however, blood insulin level drops significantly. Except for those three insulin peaks, the body is in a low-insulin state for the

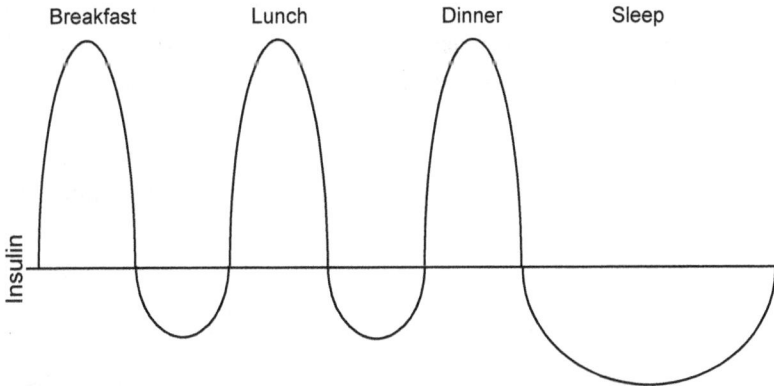

Figure 13.1. 24-hour insulin levels with a dietary pattern consisting of 3 meals a day

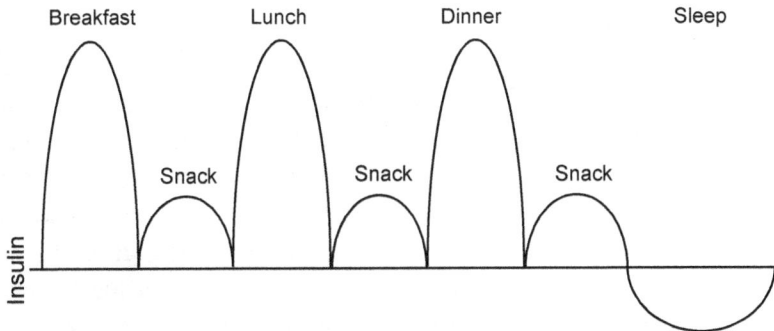

Figure 13.2. 24-hour insulin levels with a dietary pattern consisting of 6 meals a day

rest of the day; thus the risk of developing insulin resistance is negligible.

On the other hand, if you eat 6 meals a day, your body is constantly in a high-insulin state. There is a short period, exclusively in the second half of the night, when insulin levels will drop significantly (see Figure 13.2). As discussed earlier, insulin diverts nutrients into fat deposits; therefore it should be viewed as the main driving force behind obesity. The constantly high insulin levels, which are a result of a habit of continuous grazing, explain why it is nearly impossible to achieve a significant weight loss on a *6 meals a day* dietary protocol.

During low-insulin periods, the body gradually uses up its own energy deposits instead of putting the absorbed nutrients into fat storage. When exogenous glucose (the sugar from the food) runs out, glycogen from the liver and muscles will be converted into glucose. Once glycogen reserves are depleted, typically within 16 to 20 hours, body fat becomes the primary energy source. In order to maximize weight loss, our primary goal should be setting the eating window as narrow as possible. The ideal width of the eating window is about eight hours. In other words, the length of time between the first and the last meal of the day shouldn't be longer than eight hours. For example, breakfast should be served at 8 AM, lunch at noon, and dinner at 4 PM; no other meals or caloric beverages are allowed throughout the day. For those who can not accommodate a regimen of an 8 hour eating window, the time frame between the first and the last meal of the day may be extended to 10 hours. As a general rule, the narrower your eating window, the faster the weight loss. Under no circumstances should the eating window be left wider than 12 hours. A narrow eating window greatly accelerates fat burning, while long feeding periods interfere with weight loss.

THE SECOND MEAL PHENOMENON

The *second meal phenomenon* or *Staub-Traugott effect* has been known for a century. If two similar meals are followed by each other within a period of four hours, the blood sugar raising effect of the second meal will be considerably lower than of the first meal. We can take the advantage of the *second meal effect* when planning our dietary protocol. If two meals are consumed within a time period of four hours, the fattening effect of the second meal will slightly decrease.

SUMMARY

We can conclude that the question of *when to eat* is nearly as important as *what to eat*. Narrowing down the eating window of our dietary plan should be one of our top priorities. During fasting periods, the insulin production pauses and the body's sensitivity to the hormone significantly improves. Restoring the body's insulin sensitivity is the key to a successful, long-term weight management program. *Intermittent fasting* is an extremely powerful weapon in your battle against obesity.

The *American Diabetes Association* calls type-2 diabetes an incurable progressive disease that will get worse over time. Contrary to the widely-held belief, in many cases, in addition to promoting weight loss, fasting is even capable of reversing type-2 diabetes[52] .

Besides *intermittent fasting* there are two more helpful ideas that can further improve the efficiency of your weight loss. First, don't eat late at night. The same food has a less fattening effect if is consumed in the morning, rather than in the evening. Second, if two meals are followed by each other within four hours, the second meal has a less blood-sugar raising effect. This is called the *second meal phenomenon.*

14

THE IMPORTANCE OF EXERCISING

THE EXERCISE PARADOX

There are many conflicting views on the role of exercise in weight management. Proponents of the *calories in-calories out* model explain obesity merely as a caloric imbalance between energy intake and expenditure. If that were the case, in order to lose weight, the only thing you need to do would be either to reduce your caloric intake or to increase your energy expenditure. This theory is based on a series of key assumptions and has turned out to be totally wrong. Managing the energy metabolism of the human body is way more complicated than just counting calories in and calories out.

Despite the opposing views on the usefulness of working out, the exercise craze has been on the rise since the 1970s. The foundations of a multi-billion dollar fitness industry were laid on this very fragile and questionable calorie counting theory. Over the last four decades our gigantic efforts to stop the obesity epidemic have all failed; the time and money we've spent on exercising grew parallel with our body mass index.

Michelle Obama's *Let's Move!* campaign didn't lack ambition. President Obama's wife aimed to eliminate the problem of obesity within one generation. The main objectives of the program were to serve healthy food in schools and to increase the physical activity levels of the students. Providing healthier food choices for our children and involving them in sports and outdoor activities is an excellent idea, however these measures didn't really stop the rapidly increasing childhood obesity epidemic. Since 2010, when the program was launched, childhood obesity didn't decrease at all. The fact of the matter is, that despite the heroic efforts, youth obesity rates during the first 7 years of the *Let's Move!* program just kept on going up, from 16.9% to 18.5%. Why do all fitness programs fail in the long run? We will see later in this chapter, that physical exercise is an extremely inefficient way to expend energy. In addition to that, regular workouts and various outdoor activities cause us to develop a very healthy appetite, and it is nearly impossible to lose weight through physical exercise alone.

In contrast to the fitness movement, some proponents of the hormonal obesity theory argue that in the development of obesity, physical activity level makes no difference at all. Since they completely reject the *calories in-calories out model*, they believe that obesity is determined by hormonal levels only, predominantly regulated by insulin, partially by cortisol, and a few other hormones as well. Relying solely on either the caloric or the hormonal approach grossly oversimplifies the theory of obesity. The regulation of weight loss and weight gain are very complex physiological processes.

Let's take a quick look at the physiology of the human body and see how we respond to changes in our energy expenditure. The *basal metabolic rate* is the amount of energy expended by humans at rest, maintaining just the basic functions of the organs of the body. It makes up 70 percent of our daily energy expenditure. Another 10 percent of the total energy use is allocated to heat production. Only 20 percent of our energy expenditure is used for physical activities. From the *calories in-calories out* view point, being involved in strenuous physical exercise is an extremely inefficient solution to lose weight. For example, a small, 25 gram chocolate chip cookie contains 122 kcal of energy. To burn these excess calories you have to sweat in the gym for 15 minutes or walk for half an hour. It is definitely not worth it. In addition to the inefficiency of working out, there is another catch too: vigorous physical exercise and outdoor activities may ultimately lead to increased hunger. At the end of the day, instead of losing weight, you may easily end up even gaining some weight. Besides these issues, there is another problem as well. If you do your exercise in the morning, later your metabolic rate may noticeably slow down; you will be a little bit sluggish for the rest of the day and will spend less energy on other physical activities. As a result, your net energy balance will be nearly zero. In other words, according to the *calories in-calories out* model, you won't lose weight.

The *Harvard School of Public Health* did a study[53] with the participation of 538 students to determine if physical exercise leads to a negative energy balance. Researchers found that those children who participated in one hour of moderate physical activity– as a result of their increased appetite– actually consumed 99 calories more than they burned by exercising. Those who were involved in medium-level physical activity just broke even: they hardly managed to expend the extra calories they ate. Only the children who exercised vigorously were able to burn 93 calories in an hour. This experiment demonstrates the difficulty of weight loss by exercising. Following physical exercise, due to the energy compensation mechanism, our body demands us to replenish the amount of expended energy (occasionally even more) by way of extra food consumption. Instead of helping you lose weight, moderate physical activity may even result in weight gain by stimulating your appetite.

The health effect of physical education classes was assessed [54] in another study with the participation of 955 fourth grade students. The intervention group was enrolled in an extended physical education program with an additional 41 minutes of exercising each week. Children in the control group continued their regular curriculum. The physical activity level of the students was evaluated by an accelerometer (a small electronic device that detects body movements by measuring acceleration). At the end of the fourth and fifth school year, the relevant data was collected and analyzed. The results of the experiment were very controversial. The overall fitness level of the children in the intervention group turned out to be much higher, but their energy expenditure remained almost the same. Those kids who exercised harder at school, tended to be more sedentary at home. The total daily energy expenditure of boys was identical in both groups. More surprisingly, the total energy expenditure of the girls in the experimental group was even 12% lower than of those who didn't exercise that much. This is the previously mentioned energy compensation process: the body defends its default weight, preset by our internal "thermostat".

Coca Cola spent over 4 billion dollars on advertising in 2016. The company sponsors the Olympic games, soccer world championships, NASCAR, and many other important sporting events. On their website there are hundreds of articles, news updates, and interviews with popular athletes. The company built up a very strong, persuasive image that associates their products with youth, sports, mobility, and an active lifestyle. Their message suggests that in spite of the excessively high sugar content, it is ok to drink Coke, as long as you exercise and live a physically active life. Such commercials subconsciously program our minds to believe that we can get rid of the excess calories simply by exercising. It is hard to tell which one is more harmful to our health: this ideology, or the products themselves.

WHY IS EXERCISING SO IMPORTANT

From the conventional *calories in-calories out* viewpoint, physical exercise as a weight-loss tool is no better than snake oil. After exercising, as the compensatory mechanism kicks in, your metabolism will slow down or you will feel an urge to eat more. Inevitably, we come across a very important question: *Is exercising necessary at all?* I have bad news for you: the answer is definitely yes. Let's see why.

As we saw earlier, both obesity and type-2 diabetes have the same underlying cause: insulin resistance. Physical exercise significantly improves the body's insulin sensitivity through its double action mechanism. As a result of muscle contractions, GLUT-4 transporter proteins translocate to the cell surface and facilitate glucose uptake by the cells.[4] This type of glucose transport doesn't require insulin. Once the first mechanism is exhausted, then comes the second action. The second and long-lasting result of physical exercise is sensitizing the body to insulin's effects. Since the body's insulin sensitivity greatly improves, the pancreas has to secrete lower amounts of the hormone. As a result of reduced insulin levels, less energy will be stored as body fat.

Although a caloric imbalance is not the main cause of obesity, in certain individuals, a moderate weight reduction can still be achieved by participating in physical exercise alone. However, care should be taken not to overeat, because the benefits of our increased physical activity level can be easily lost by increased food intake.

Regular physical exercise helps you break down fat tissue and build up new lean muscle mass. Muscle tissue has a higher metabolic rate than fat. Even if your body weight doesn't change, you will still burn more energy.

In addition to these health benefits, a physically active lifestyle greatly reduces the risk factors for a wide range of life-threatening diseases such as coronary heart disease, stroke, thrombosis, type-2 diabetes and cancer. Regular physical exercise also plays an important role in the prevention of arthritis, osteoporosis, dementia and depression.

SUMMARY

Participating in regular physical exercise is a very simple, but extremely powerful tool in the prevention of several chronic diseases. Although the direct caloric effect of exercising on weight loss is very limited, regular physical activities greatly increase the body's insulin sensitivity. By restoring our normal insulin sensitivity, the pancreas has to produce less insulin. Lower insulin levels protect us from obesity and stimulate weight loss as well. Regular physical exercise is capable of normalizing our insulin levels for several hours, leaving a certain level of protection for up to a day after exercising.

For every healthy individual, half an hour of medium-intensity physical exercise is recommended at least five or six times a week. In order to enjoy all the benefits of these protective effects, each session should contain at least 25-30 minutes of *continuous* exercising. On the top of our regular exercise, being involved in extra physical activities is fine, but it has just a minimal extra health benefit.

15

THE FORMULA FOR WEIGHT LOSS

THE CHICKEN OR THE EGG DEBATE

In *Part 2* of this book we've reviewed the most common theories of obesity: *genetics, fattening carbohydrates, calories in-calories out, the fat theory,* and *the hormonal obesity theory,* including the *carbohydrate-insulin model.* All of these theories contain some elements of truth, with one exception: the fat theory turned out to be totally wrong. Fats are not fattening per se. A given number of calories from fats make you definitely less obese than the same amount of energy taken from carbohydrates.

Today's mainstream science and medicine is dominated by the *calories in-calories out* theory. The *carbohydrate-insulin model* is the most popular alternative theory, especially among the proponents of the low-carb diets. The simplified diagrams of these theories were shown on Figure 10.2. and Figure 12.1 in the previous chapters.

The *conventional model* of obesity considers energy intake and expenditure independent of each other (see Figure 15.1). Overeating and physical inactivity increases the amounts of circulating metabolic fuels (glucose, lipids). The excess nutrients will be deposited into fat tissue. Obesity is the *consequence* of a caloric imbalance. In order to lose weight, the only thing you need to do is either eat less or exercise more. This approach has been proven to be totally wrong. Millions of dieters who meticulously follow this advice fail each year.

The alternative theory is called the *carbohydrate-insulin model* (see Figure 15.2). Refined carbohydrates cause hyperinsulinemia. Higher than normal insulin levels promote the deposit of calories into fat cells, ultimately leading to obesity. Since calories are diverted into fat storage, the rest of the body is in starvation mode. Energy deprivation leads to increased hunger, fatigue and physical inactivity.

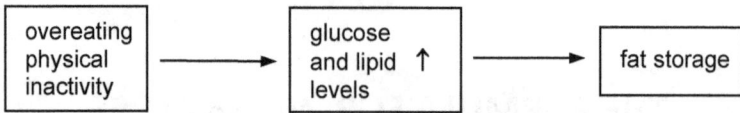

Figure 15.1. Conventional model of obesity

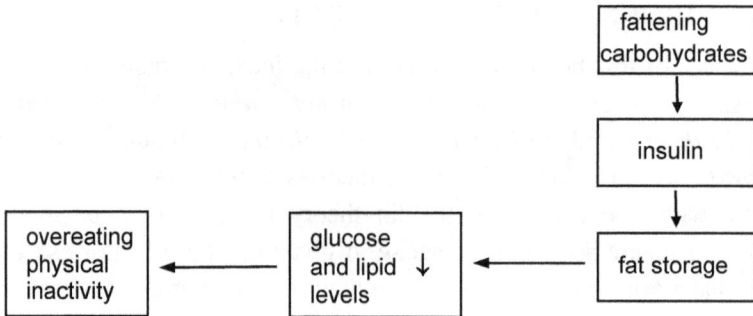

Figure 15.2. Carbohydrate-insulin model of obesity

Overeating is the *consequence*, NOT the cause of obesity. In the second chart, the arrows point in the opposite direction compared to in the first chart. The conventional theory is also known as the *push model*, and the *carbohydrate-insulin theory* as the *pull model* of obesity.

Skeptics may think that the alternative model of obesity is something new, not well documented, and lacks all the scientific evidence. This is not the case, however. The basic idea of the alternative theory was first proposed in 1908 by German scientist *Gustav von Bergmann*, and then taken up by the Czech-Austrian researcher *Julius Bauer*. Bergmann discovered that in certain areas of the body, fat cells accumulate excessive amounts of fat, while depriving other regions of nutrients, leading to starvation. He called the phenomenon *lipophilia*. In 1929 Bauer wrote: "Like a malignant tumor or like the fetus" ... "the abnormal lipophilic tissue seizes on foodstuffs, even in the case of undernutrition." In his 1941 paper, Bauer said: "The current energy theory of obesity, which considers only an imbalance between intake of food and expenditure of energy, is unsatisfactory." As Germany lost World War II, the scientific evidence supporting the alternative theory of obesity also got lost, until it was re-discovered at the end of the 20ᵗʰ century. In the meantime, the junk-food-industry-sponsored mainstream nutrition scientists kept on bombarding us with their slogan: "A calorie is a calorie". According to their theory, all calories are identical and there is no difference between "bad" calories and "good" calories.

Although the *carbohydrate-insulin theory* seems to be the most accurate one of the previously-mentioned models to explain obesity, it is still incomplete and leaves some unanswered questions. Critics often cite that "Overeating causes obesity". That's right. On the other hand, there is also a compensatory mechanism. Overfeeding studies show, that when the protocol ends, body weight tends to return to near baseline[55]. We should keep in mind however, that subjects typically don't lose the full amount of weight they have gained, just a portion of it. In other words, the compensatory effect is just partial.

In addition to its incompleteness, there were some minor discrepancies also found in the *carbohydrate-insulin model*. The theory proposes that due to the hyperactivity of fat cells, low blood glucose and lipid levels will occur within 2.5 to 5 hours after food consumption. However, obesity is typically associated with high levels of these metabolic fuels. According to *David S. Ludwig*, low blood glucose and lipid levels typically occur during the dynamic stage of obesity development only.[56] In the later stage of obesity however, circulating metabolic fuel concentrations rise. The level of blood glucose and lipids provide only an indirect and imperfect indication of cellular metabolism. Circulating metabolic fuel levels doesn't diminish the validity of the theory. The *carbohydrate-insulin model* shouldn't be viewed as a complete theory that gives an exhaustive explanation to the causes of obesity, rather, just a conceptual framework for understanding the etiology of obesity.

THE NEW MODEL OF OBESITY

My greatest concern about the existing theories is that they all claim to be the only true explanation of the problem of obesity. This reductionist approach turned out to be totally wrong. Obesity has not just one single cause but multiple causes. The objective of my research was to combine these viable theories into a single framework for modeling the causes of obesity. The hormonal concept of obesity is a good starting point. Figure 15.3 shows the diagram of the new model of obesity that is built on the foundations of the hormonal theory. The rest of this chapter explains the role of each factor in the development of obesity.

GENETIC FACTORS

Many people say "I can not lose weight, obesity is in my genes." If this applies to you, I have to say you are not the only one. About 70% of the whole population is prone to obesity. Although genetics is an important part of the equation, genes by themselves do not cause obesity (except for a few extremely rare cases). For example, possible genetic causes may include leptin gene mutation or Prader-Willi syndrome. Although Prader-Willi syndrome is the most common genetic cause of morbid obesity in children, it occurs only once in every 25,000 births. Considering the fact that in industrialized countries, nearly one third of the population is obese and another third is in the overweight category, only a negligible number of these people have a primary genetic cause for their weight problem. Most of us are prone to obesity, however it is our lifestyle and the environment that activates those genes and make us obese. The *Inherited Obesity* chapter of this book discusses the genetic background of obesity in more detail.

INSULIN IS THE MAIN CULPRIT

Foods rich in easily digestible carbohydrates, especially in sugar and starch, produce *hyperinsulinemia*, a condition with higher than normal levels of insulin in the blood. Elevated insulin levels promote the deposit of calories in fat cells instead of utilizing the energy in

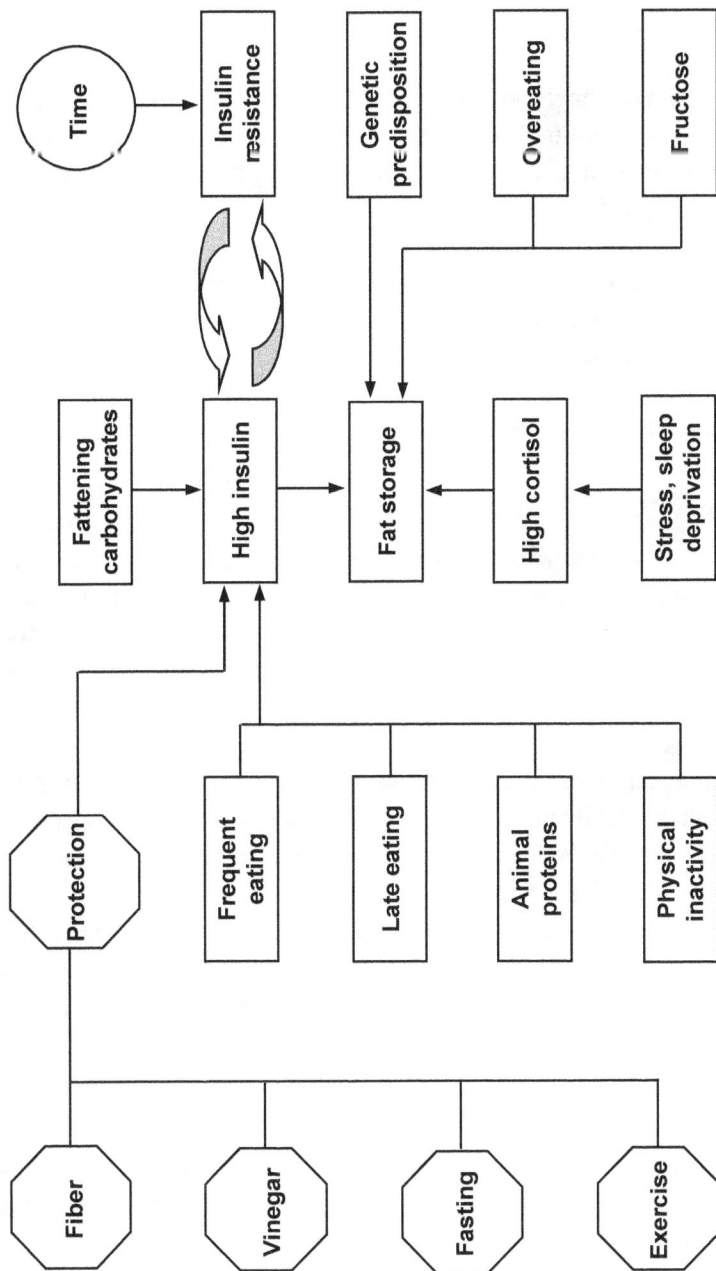

Figure 15.3. The new model of obesity. Protective factors are shown in octagons, risks are in rectangles.

lean tissues, ultimately leading to obesity. The *Hormonal Obesity* chapter of this book discusses in more detail, how hormones affect obesity.

People who have been obese for most of their lives may find it extremely difficult to lose weight. In contrast, those who have become obese just recently, can get rid of their excess pounds with considerably less effort. How is all that possible? Over time, obese people tend to develop insulin resistance. The longer the duration of obesity, the worse insulin resistance gets. As obesity progresses, the cells of the human body gradually become desensitized to insulin's effect, causing high blood sugar levels. As a result, the pancreas secretes more insulin. Higher blood insulin levels further exacerbate insulin resistance, forming a vicious cycle.

CORTISOL

After insulin, *cortisol* is the second most important hormone closely related to the development of obesity. In response to long-term stress exposure, adrenal glands secrete a steroid hormone called cortisol. This hormone stimulates glycogen storage in the liver and the formation of *visceral fat* deposits. Visceral fat surrounds internal organs, located deep in the *peritonium*. Excessive amounts of visceral fat cause abdominal obesity. Abdominal fat is substantially different from subcutaneous fat (fat located under the skin); abdominal obesity is a serious risk factor for cardiovascular disease. Long term stress exposure may lead to obesity. In addition to stimulating cortisol production, stress also increases appetite. Reducing our stress level is not easy; however, getting an adequate amount of sleep may significantly lower our stress and cortisol levels.

THE ESSENCE OF TIME

We've read in the *What to Eat vs. When to Eat* chapter that the question *when to eat* is almost as important as w*hat to eat*. Frequent eating and snacking between meals keeps our insulin level constantly high. As discussed earlier, insulin is the main driving force behind obesity. Narrowing down the eating window (the period of time between the first and last meal of the day) should be one of our top priorities in our weight-loss strategy.

In addition to reducing the length of the eating period, there is another useful tip that can further improve the efficiency of your weight-loss method. The physiological processes in our body follow a daily rhythm. Researchers found that the insulin sensitivity of the human cells is better in the morning than later during the day. In other words, the same food has less fattening effect in the morning than in the evening. Therefore, night eating and snacking should be avoided.

OVEREATING

Although we previously showed that the *calories in-calories out* approach cannot give you a full explanation of the development of obesity, calories still do matter. Some proponents of the *hormonal obesity model* try to convince us that calories don't make any difference at all. Both the concept of *calorie-denial* and of *calorie counting* are equally wrong. It is an unquestionable fact that in case of most individuals, overeating leads to obesity. Basically, what causes the confusion is that there are several compensatory mechanisms interfering with the *calories in-calories out model*. Some of these effects may stimulate weight loss while others promote weight gain. For example, reducing caloric intake slows down the metabolic rate. This is why all calorie restricted diets fail in the long run. Conversely, if you eat more than usual, you will also burn more energy. As a result, fewer calories will end up as body fat, than expected by the calorie-counting method. Another confounding factor is that foods with various glycemic indexes have different effects on your blood sugar and insulin level as well, thus they have quite different fattening effects. Not all calories are alike.

Nevertheless, we can conclude that the amount of consumed calories is not the primary cause of obesity, however overeating definitely leads to obesity.

OTHER FACTORS

Fructose naturally occurs in fruits at a moderate concentration. This sugar is also widely used by the junk food industry: it is the main ingredient of most sugar-sweetened beverages and is frequently added to processed foods. Manufacturers prefer using fructose in their products, because it has a more intensely sweet taste than any other sugars and it can be cheaply produced from corn. A fructose-rich diet has several adverse health effects: fructose increases the risk of developing insulin resistance, raises triglyceride levels and may cause non-alcoholic fatty liver disease.

Excessive meat consumption is also a risk factor for obesity. Plant proteins have a different amino acid ratio than animal proteins do. Plant proteins trigger a less intense insulin response than animal proteins and have a less fattening effect.[57]

PROTECTIVE EFFECTS

Personally, I would call fiber man's best friend, at least from a nutritional point of view. Dietary fiber has numerous health benefits, including reducing the risk of developing some cancers, hyperlipidemia, hypertension, coronary heart disease and type-2 diabetes. Dietary fibers slow down the absorption rate of carbohydrates and reduce the post-meal insulin response. As a result of lower insulin levels, less energy is deposited in fat cells. Fibers also delay gastric emptying which results in an extended feeling of fullness.

Vinegar, this food ingredient that has been consumed since ancient times, is our second best friend. The main health benefit of vinegar is reducing the glucose and insulin responses following a carbohydrate meal. Due to its insulin lowering effect, adding vinegar to our daily diet is a very powerful weight-loss tool.

In *The Importance of Exercising* chapter we saw that living a physically active lifestyle not only helps you lose weight but also prevents numerous chronic diseases. Regarding the role of physical exercise in weight loss, there is a very common misconception. Some experts argue that you can simply not lose weight by exercising. The role of exercising in weight loss is much more complex. Although it's a scientific fact that working out is an extremely inefficient way of expending energy, exercising still has many indirect health benefits. Participating in regular physical activities greatly improves the body's insulin sensitivity and decreases insulin production. Restoring normal insulin levels protects us from obesity and stimulates weight loss. Conversely, a predominantly sedentary lifestyle is one of the major risk factors for becoming obese.

Fasting is the most powerful one of all the dietary measures. You can read more about the topic of fasting and find a detailed practical guide in the *What to Eat vs. When to Eat chapter*. Let me illustrate how this simple but extremely efficient tool helps you lose weight. Obviously, there is zero caloric intake while fasting. Although the food consumption during the next meal or two following a fasting may be slightly higher than normal, the total amount of consumed calories on a fasting day and a following feeding day is still less than usual. Fasting definitely results in a negative energy balance. More importantly, in addition to the reduced caloric intake, fasting significantly improves the body's insulin sensitivity. As a result, the pancreas has to produce lower quantities of the hormone. Lower insulin levels result in a less fattening effect. Fasting helps you break out of the vicious cycle of insulin resistance that is the main cause of obesity, in the case of most individuals.

Many dieters have already experienced the so-called "thermostat effect". Our body desperately defends our preset weight. For example, if you eat less, instead of losing weight, your body will switch into an energy-saving mode. Your metabolism will slow down and you will end up burning fewer calories. There is an invisible mechanism that keeps our body weight the same in the long run, just like the thermostat regulates the temperature of your house. Besides bariatric surgery, fasting is the only available method that is capable of resetting your inner "weight thermostat".

SUMMARY

In this chapter, we saw that the question of *what causes obesity* is way more complex than previously thought. Calories, nutrients, fasting, hormones, genetics, your lifestyle and even the duration of obesity all have a significant impact on your body weight. Caloric intake is just one of the several terms of this very complex equation.

PART

THREE

BAD MEDICINE

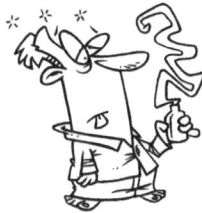

PART

THREE

16

"BIG BILL" ROCKEFELLER THE FRAUD

HOW THE CORRUPTION OF HEALTHCARE BEGAN

To investigate the roots of the corruption in our modern-day healthcare system, we need to go back one and a half centuries in time. The billionaire John D. Rockefeller's father, *William Avery Rockefeller*, also known as "Big Bill" was a traveling salesman of quack medicines made up mostly of crude oil and alcohol. Although he never received any form of medical training, he had advertising signs saying "Dr. William A. Rockefeller, the Celebrated Cancer Specialist, Here for One Day Only. All cases of Cancer Cured unless too far gone and then they can be greatly benefited".[58] For a cancer treatment Rockefeller charged $25; that sum was two months wages for a farm worker. Big Bill had practically no moral code. He loaned money to farmers at twelve per cent interest. Rockefeller purposely lent to borrowers who were not able to pay, so he could foreclose on their farms.

There were several court cases against Big Bill. He was charged with a whole range of serious crimes including bigamy, raping a girl hired in his household, and horse theft. To avoid prosecution, Big Bill moved with his family to Cleveland, Ohio, outside the New York court's jurisdiction.

Big Bill often cheated and even tricked his own sons as much as he could, to "make them sharp". That was the father's main goal. This is the family background of John D. Rockefeller, who became the world's richest person in his time. It is well-known that history is always written by the winners. After becoming rich, John D. Rockefeller would do anything to maintain a positive image of a philanthropic business man who started his career as a 16-year-old accountant clerk boy and made his fortune by honest, hard work. Big

Bill's past was one of the Rockefellers best kept dark secrets. In 1900, *Joseph Pulitzer*–the publisher and one of the most desperate critics of Rockefeller's methods – offered an $8,000 award for information on the whereabouts of Rockefeller's father who was hiding under a false name. Despite the journalists' significant efforts to find him, they failed to track him down before he died. Big Bill's story was published only years after his death.

At the time John D. Rockefeller died in 1937, his total assets were estimated at $1.4 billion which equaled one and a half percent of the United States' GDP at that time. John D. Rockefeller made his never-before-seen fortune by building a monopoly of the oil industry during the late 19th century and early 20th century. As his wealth grew, he gradually acquired interests in banking, shipping, mining, railroads, and other industries as well.

Readers may ask the question: How is the corruption of our healthcare system related to the Rockefellers? Well, it is an undeniable fact that modern healthcare greatly relies on petroleum. For example, the fuel to transport patients, the raw materials for numerous pharmaceuticals, plastics and medical supplies all require massive amounts of petroleum products. A hundred years ago, John D. Rockefeller had a vision to transform medicine through replacing well-established traditional methods with allopathic medicine dedicated to surgery and the heavy use of drugs. During the 20th century, the Rockefellers gradually built up a global, multi-billion dollar pharmaceutical industry, which became the precursor of the today's "monster", often referred to as *Big Pharma*. In the following chapters, I will explain how the Rockefeller empire corrupted the healthcare system and took control of the medical schools of the United States.

17

RISE OF THE BIG PHARMA

MONOPOLIZING THE MEDICAL EDUCATION SYSTEM

The *American Medical Association* (AMA), was founded in 1847, to "promote the art and science of medicine and the betterment of public health". Unfortunately by today, the AMA has become no more than just an extension of the powerful pharmaceutical lobby. Let me give you a short insight on how Western medicine got corrupted over the past two centuries.

During the 19th century, there were two dominant trends in medicine: allopathic and traditional medicine. Doctors practicing allopathic medicine heavily relied on the new concept of using drugs and surgery to treat diseases (or just to suppress the symptoms), just like today's Western medicine. In contrast, traditional medicine used various methods that were passed on from one generation to another. Both sides have their shortfalls. Traditional medicine is often mixed with quackery and pseudo-science. On the other hand, allopathic medicine is supposed to be based on strict scientific principles. However, the fact that allopathy heavily relies on drugs and surgery gave a great opportunity to the newly emerging chemical industry to take control of modern medicine. Back in the middle of the 19th century, doctors practicing allopathic medicine were still in the minority compared to those working with traditional methods. A few decades later, after monopolizing the American oil industry and acquiring interests in many other sectors as well, the Rockefellers had a plan to expand their business to dominate the whole pharmaceutical industry as well. As a first step, the Rockefeller empire had to take over the entire medical education system of the United States. They financially supported those medical schools that integrated the principles of allopathic medicine in their curriculum. New generations of doctors were raised to rely solely on drugs and surgery, and to despise traditional methods.

In 1904, the American Medical Association formed the *Council on Medical Education* (CME), whose objective was to reform the entire American medical education system. In 1910, with support from the Rockefellers and the Carnegie Foundation, *Abraham Flexner* published a survey on the existing medical schools in the United States and Canada, which later became famously known as the *Flexner Report*. In 1902, one of the first foundations established by the Rockefeller family was the *General Education Board*. By 1960, the Board's initial 94 million dollars and the conditional matches totaled 600 million dollars, which was committed to funding medical schools.[59] Typical of the Rockefellers, the privatization of the American medical education system appeared to be as a great gesture of their generosity and philanthropy. However, the Rockefellers' real intention was to gradually expand their interests into the pharmaceutical industry. In order to achieve their goal they had to take control of the whole medical education system of the United States. Those institutions who received grants from the Rockefellers, were told what to teach to the medical students and what curricula they had to adopt. Drug and surgery-based medicine was the only correct approach; other alternatives were not tolerated and were labeled as "quackery" or "charlatanism". Medical schools that taught other approaches besides the excessive use of drugs and surgery fell short of necessary funding. The non-compliant schools were quickly forced out of business.

To grab public attention, Rockefeller's "matching funds" formula was a brilliant idea. Although only a quarter of donations came from the Rockefellers, they took all the public credit for donations and maintained the control over the funds as well, since they were the largest single contributor. Over the course of the following decades Big Pharma established its non-profit shadow-organizations such as the *American Cancer Society, American Heart Association, American Diabetes Association, and the American Lung Association* - the list goes on and on. After developing a monopoly of the oil industry, the Rockefellers successfully privatized the entire medical education system too. Since then, several generations of doctors already grew up who were taught the exclusive use of drugs and surgery. The negative impact of excessive drug usage on our health is unprecedented. By now, 45% of the U.S. population uses prescription drugs. *Peter Gøtzsche*, the co-founder of the *Cochrane Collaboration*, estimates that prescribed medication is the third most common cause of death globally after heart disease and cancer. Let's conclude with one of Rockefeller's favorite sayings: "I don't want a nation of thinkers, I want a nation of workers."

FAILURE OF THE HEALTH CARE SYSTEM

Americans' health is worse than ever. Among the industrialized countries, the United States has the lowest life expectancy. Two thirds of Americans are obese or overweight. As of 2012, about half of all adults had one or more chronic health conditions. In 2016, 4.4 billion prescriptions were dispensed. Nearly 70% of the *middle aged population* regularly takes prescription drugs. The same year, Americans spent over $328 billion on prescriptions. Since the year 2000, this amount has nearly tripled. Although the United States has the highest per capita health expenditure in the world, the overall health of Americans is nearly the worst among the industrialized countries.

WHY ARE DRUGS SO EXPENSIVE?

In 2017, the U.S. *Food and Drug Administration* (FDA) approved 46 new drugs, the highest number in over two decades. Curious readers may ask the question: are new drugs necessarily better than the old ones used for decades? "Why change what works?" , "If it isn't broken, don't fix it!" - These are old sayings containing a lot of truth and wisdom.

Dr. *Marcia Angell*, the former editor of *The New England Journal of Medicine* says when submitting a new product to FDA for approval, pharmaceutical companies don't have to compare the new drugs to existing drugs to test the efficiency to treat a given health condition.[60] They just need to compare the new drug with a placebo. The only thing they have to prove is that the new drug is slightly better than nothing. If new drugs are not necessarily better than existing ones, then why do pharmaceutical companies spend billions of dollars on the development of new products when existing drugs are available at a fraction of the cost?

Selling prescription drugs is an incredibly lucrative business. In 2016, worldwide prescription drug sales totaled 768 billion dollars. This astronomical amount of money is 8 times more than *Bill Gates'* total assets. For example, if Gates sold everything he owned, and decided to pay for people's medications, he would run out of money after 6 weeks and his whole fortune would be gone.

Returning to the original question, why do pharmaceutical companies spend billions of dollars on new drugs? The answer may sound a little bit surprising: for more profit. Upon the discovery of a new drug, the first step is to have it patented. In most countries, patents are valid for 20 years. During the lifetime of a patent, the inventor has an exclusive right to produce and sell the product. Since patent laws provide a monopoly for inventors, they can sell their product for as high a price as they want. This explains why prescription drugs are so expensive. However, after 20 years, when the patent expires, the intellectual property becomes a *public domain* and anybody has the right to produce the drug without the permission of the inventor. Within a short period of time, competitors will offer a generic version of the same drug at a fraction of the original price. This is the point when the inventor usually comes up with a new drug at a much higher price instead of competing with other manufacturers. However, the previously mentioned period of 20 years is practically much shorter. After patent registration, manufacturers need to get the new drug approved by the FDA, which takes a long time, usually a couple of years. The end result is that the lifetime of a new drug is significantly less than 20 years. Manufacturers need to squeeze the maximum profit from their products over the course of the remaining time; this drives up drug prices even further.

BIG PHARMA'S SALES AGENTS

The sale of prescription medication is definitely the most profitable segment of the whole pharmaceutical industry. Since those drugs can

only be prescribed by medical professionals, pharmaceutical companies have traditionally focused their marketing activities on doctors
and pharmacists. Although, in most countries physicians are not allowed to receive any kind of compensation from drug manufacturers
for prescribing certain drugs, doctors have unwittingly become the
top selling agents of the pharmaceutical industry. Since Big Pharma
has been controlling the whole medical education system in the
Western world for a century, several generations of doctors have
already been raised on the principles of allopathic medicine that
heavily relies on the use of drugs, radiation, and surgery.

It is extremely difficult to prove if a doctor receives illegal kick-
backs from drug or medical device companies. We can assume that
this is not happening very often in the medical community. However,
dinners, traveling, conferences, and research grants are typically paid
by drug manufacturers. In 2017, for the first time in Canada, ten of
the country's largest pharmaceutical companies voluntarily disclosed
the payments that were made to doctors. For example, in 2016 *Merck*
paid over 7 million dollars and *Roche* more than 6 million to healthcare professionals.

In addition to such legally permissible methods to bribe healthcare
professionals, pharmaceutical companies found a new way to increase their sales figures: they often promote their products directly
to consumers through advertising campaigns in the public media. In
many countries, patients are regularly reminded to go buy a certain
drug or to refill their medication.

BIG PHARMA GOES TO CHINA

China, due to its huge market size, has been particularly attracting
foreign investors since the 1980s. An interesting fact is that Rockefellers' Big Pharma discovered the endless business potential of the
East Asian country more than a century ago, decades earlier than
when the transnational corporations first started investing in China.
In 1914, the Rockefeller Foundation established the *China Medical
Board*, with the intention of promoting Western medicine in Asian
countries. The board continuously operated until 1951, when the
communist regime banned the organization. Over the years, the

China Medical Board has supported 28 medical schools throughout the country.

By the end of the 19th century, the concept of *traditional Chinese medicine* stood in opposition to Western medicine. Before that, most of the Chinese doctors were open to both traditional and Western medicine. By the 1920s however, things started to change. As a result of increasing Western influence, the concept of traditional Chinese medicine was viewed as outdated by medical practitioners.

One of the country's most famous institutions, The *Peking Union Medical College* was founded in 1906. A few years later, Rockefellers' Medical Board took control of the college and assumed full support of the school, having previously acquired the property. Over the course of the following years, the Rockefellers' gradually extended their influence to the whole Chinese medical school system. Traditional Chinese medicine became a political issue. Despite 3000 years of existence, traditional medicine lost its dominant position and was replaced with drug and surgery-based practices. This didn't happen because Western medicine was necessarily superior to the traditional methods, but rather medicine was part of the conflict between Chinese and Western culture.

BIG PHARMA KILLS MORE PEOPLE THAN ILLICIT DRUGS

The use of illicit drugs is an enormous, growing problem throughout the United States. According to the *National Institute on Drug Abuse*, In 2015, illegal drugs caused the death of more than 21,800 people in the U.S.[61] During the past fifteen years, the number of deaths has increased four times. Many people are not aware of the fact however, that Big Pharma kills even more people than illicit drugs do. In 2015, prescription drugs caused the death of over 29,700 people in the United States. Similarly to illicit drugs, the increase is almost four times since 2000.

Medieval doctors sometimes treated their patients with poisonous materials such as mercury, antimony or lead. Today, the medical use of these dangerous substances belongs in the past, however modern allopathic medicine still uses a whole range of various highly toxic materials. *Cytotoxic drugs*, widely used in cancer treatment, but also for rheumatoid arthritis and multiple sclerosis, contain chemicals which are toxic to cells, preventing their replication or growth. These medicines often cause life-threatening side effects. Although chemotherapeutic drugs can be used successfully in the treatment of certain cancers like leukemia, in the case of many other cancers chemotherapy may be absolutely useless. *Cancer overtreatment* has received much recent media attention. There are certain ethical concerns regarding the system of how physicians prescribe cancer drugs. As previously discussed, in the United States, it is illegal for doctors to receive any form of compensation from drug manufacturers for prescriptions. However, in the case of cancer medications, there is a loophole left in the system: physicians are allowed to purchase cancer drugs at wholesale prices and resell them to their patients, generating massive profits.[62] In this case, doctors literally become Big Pharma's top salespeople.

In addition to the health risks of drug overconsumption, there are numerous serious environmental concerns as well. Manufacturing plants consume energy and produce massive amounts of toxic waste. Drug residues emptied from our bodies contaminate water supply. A vast array of pharmaceuticals - including antibiotics, mood stabilizers, and sex hormones have been found in the drinking water of at least 41 million Americans.[63] Regular water treatment plants can not handle drug residues.

SUMMARY

We saw in this chapter that at the beginning of the 20th century, the powerful pharmaceutical lobby successfully privatized the whole medical school system of the Western world. Since then, several generations of doctors already grew up who were taught the exclusive use of drugs and surgery to treat diseases. Although the vast majority of our modern-day ailments is preventable by simply adopting a healthy lifestyle, few people really pay attention to prevention. It is more profitable for today's Western medicine to suppress the symptoms of our diseases with expensive drugs and keep us on medication for as long as we live.

18

CORRUPTED SCIENCE

TOBACCO SCIENCE

The term *tobacco science* is synonymous with falsification or biased reporting of scientific data favoring a particular industry's agenda. The *Council for Tobacco Research* was formed by American tobacco companies in 1954, to fund "independent" scientific research to determine whether there is a link between smoking and lung cancer. In those days, there were still some skeptics who disputed the detrimental effects of smoking tobacco. One of them was *Dr. Henry Garland*, an internationally well-known radiologist, and another skeptic was *Dr. Ian MacDonald*, a renowned cancer surgeon. *Garland* and *MacDonald* had a mission to prove that smoking has no harmful health effects at all. MacDonald's famous saying was "A pack a day keeps lung cancer away". Ironically, both doctors' lives ended tragically. Dr. Garland, who had been a chain smoker since his childhood, died of lung cancer. Dr. MacDonald burned to death in bed in a fire started by his cigarette.

ONLY THE POSITIVE RESULTS ARE PUBLISHED

In the previous chapter, we saw how *Big Pharma* took over the entire medical school system of the Western world. In addition to that, the powerful pharmaceutical lobby controls scientific research and literature as well.

The Lancet is one of the most prestigious medical journals. *Richard Horton*, the chief editor of the paper said in 2015: "Much of the scientific literature, perhaps half, may simply be untrue" … "science has taken a turn towards darkness".[64]*Arnold Relman*, a Harvard professor and former editor of the *New England Journal of*

Medicine, heavily criticized the corruption of healthcare and medical research:

"The medical profession is being bought by the pharmaceutical industry, not only in terms of the practice of medicine, but also in terms of teaching and research" ... "The academic institutions of this country are allowing themselves to be the paid agents of the pharmaceutical industry. I think it's disgraceful".[65]

Medical journals play a central role in scientific research. For authors, publishing in a prestigious journal is crucial in order to obtain funding and help them in their career advancement. For pharmaceutical companies, published research papers confirming the efficiency of a certain drug, greatly increases their sales and drives up stock prices. Journal editors have enormous power. They determine the content of their paper, what articles will be published or rejected, and they write editorials as well. Big Pharma is well aware of that. From time to time, drug companies pay considerable amounts of money to medical journals to publish studies favorable towards their products. A large number of clinical trials are funded by pharmaceutical companies. Not surprisingly, typically the only trials that are published are the ones that support the benefits of a particular drug. The results of negative outcomes are hardly released.

Using the *Open Payments* database, researchers investigated how much money medical journals received from pharmaceutical and medical device manufacturers in 2014.[66] Half of the editors of the 52 most influential medical journals were paid some form of compensation. On average, editors each received $27,564 from the industry. In the general payments category, the editor of the *Journal of the American College of Cardiology* was paid the highest amount, $475,072; the editor of *Diabetes Care* received $212,426 in the form of research payments.

Besides Big Pharma, there is another major player: the food industry, which is having an enormous impact on research, especially within the field of nutrition science. Similarly to the pharmaceutical industry, food manufacturers fund clinical trials too. We run into the same problem of publication bias in both cases. The journals will only publish those papers which favor their sponsors and meet their expectations. However, in case of clinical trials preceding the approval of a new drug, the documents first have to be submitted to government agencies. Results of unpublished trials are still available for researchers. After considering both published and unpublished results, a publication bias in systematic reviews can be estimated by the number of positive and negative results. On the other hand, unpublished data from nutritional studies are not available.

The credibility of industry-sponsored studies is always very questionable. Investigators with a conflict of interest are more likely to arrive at positive conclusions while suppressing negative results. To ensure the integrity of clinical research, a full disclosure of financial interests should be a mandatory element of every single clinical trial.

Let's see a concrete example. These days, nobody would dispute the fact that the consumption of sugar-sweetened beverages plays a major role in today's obesity epidemic. A systematic review of several clinical trials was published in a medical journal. The paper concluded that the consumption of sugary drinks has no effect on body mass index.[67] If we read the fine print, we will see that the study was sponsored by the largest junk food companies including Coca Cola, PepsiCo and McDonald's. It greatly reminds me of our first story, where tobacco manufacturers hired scientists to prove that smoking has no harmful health effects at all. The results of those industry-sponsored studies can not be considered as scientific evidence.

19

CHOLESTEROL HYSTERIA

MASS HYSTERIA

Until the beginning of the 20th century, coronary heart disease was still very uncommon. After World War II however, along with fast paced economic growth, the prevalence rate of heart disease had exponentially increased. By the 1960s, heart disease became the most common cause of death in the industrialized world. Countries spent hundreds of millions of dollars to find the cause of the deadliest epidemic of the 20th century. Governments and health authorities, under the pressure from the public, needed to find a culprit for the most devastating disease of the century. Dietary fat was an excellent candidate. Starting from the 1950s and 60s, more and more studies were published claiming that fat consumption is one of the major risk factors for coronary heart disease. Later in this chapter we will see how the massive amount of "scientific evidence" was manufactured to support this theory.

The *lipid hypothesis* is a term referring to the assumption that high blood cholesterol causes heart disease. It has been the most widely-held view among mainstream scientists since the 1960s. As a matter of fact, there is just a moderate correlation between blood cholesterol levels and coronary heart disease, and this relationship is much weaker than previously thought. However, over the course of the following decades, a multi-billion-dollar business was built upon this very fragile theory. The cholesterol hysteria kept the healthcare system busy and generated billions of dollars of revenue for the pharmaceutical and food industries.

Mainstream media played a major role in leading to mass hysteria about dietary fat. Over the last few decades, hardly a day goes by without the headline news, articles, books or blogs constantly reminding us to avoid dietary fat. The whole society is in a constant state of hysteria. The most absurd statement ever was made by *David Kritchevsky*, the renowned biochemist: "In America, we no longer fear God or the communists, but we fear fat".

DR. ANICHKOV AND THE BUNNY RABBITS

Ancel Keys is the name of the man responsible for starting the whole anti-fat campaign and cholesterol hysteria, in the early 1950s. However, in order to understand the entire story, we need to go back to the days of the Russian tsars'. *Nikolai Nikolaevich Anichkov*, a young medical student in St. Petersburg became interested in his professor's, Dr. Ignatowski's, work. Ignatowski proposed that rabbits might develop atherosclerosis after eating non-vegetarian food, including meat and eggs. After graduation, Anichkov continued studying the disease and many years later became an internationally renowned expert of coronary atherosclerosis. From the mid-1950s, several cholesterol-induced atherosclerosis experiments were done worldwide, by using Anichkov's technique. The results were controversial. Some laboratories used other animals instead of rabbits, such as rats or dogs. Cholesterol consumption in species other than rabbits failed to induce atherosclerosis. Rabbits are strictly vegetarian animals and normally have zero cholesterol intake and a very low fat intake. The rabbit model of atherosclerosis turned out to be completely irrelevant to human disease.

ANCEL KEYS' "DOCTORED" DIAGRAM

In the early 1950s, the former marine biologist, *Ancel Keys* came up with a similarly strange theory that coronary heart disease is caused by fat consumption. Back in those days, before the outbreak of the cholesterol hysteria, Keys was often ridiculed for his bold idea. The first time in 1953, Ancel Keys, in his lecture, presented the infamous diagram at a symposium at *Mt. Sinai Hospital*.[68] In the age group of men, 55-59, the graph exhibits a nearly linear, very strong correlation between fat consumption and heart disease. Figure 19.1 shows the relationship between dietary fat intake (percentage of total energy) and the heart disease death rates in the *arbitrarily selected* six countries (For those who are statistically inclined, r=0.96 p=0.002). The diagram is very persuasive and it looks almost perfect, but there is a problem. Keys cherry-picked six countries: Japan, Italy, England, Australia, Canada and the United States. There were data available from 22 countries in total, but our expert in oceanography simply ignored the rest of the countries.

Two prominent biostatisticians, *Jacob Yerushalmy* and *Herman Hilleboe* were not very impressed by the biased results. In 1957, they published a paper on the relationship between dietary fat intake and heart disease, with the participation of 22 countries in total. The study included every single country where sufficient data was available at that point. This time, just a moderate correlation was found (r=0.51) between fat consumption and heart disease. See Figure 19.2. It should be noted however, that correlation doesn't necessarily mean causal relationship. For example, statisticians found that there is a positive correlation between ice cream sales and drowning accidents. Does ice cream cause the death of swimmers? Not really. There is a *confounder factor*: the hot weather. On warm summer days, more ice cream is sold, and more people go swimming. Therefore, more of them drown in lakes and rivers. The same principle applies if we compare the fat consumption and heart disease prevalence rates of various countries. There are many *confounder factors*: the economic situation, health care system, lifestyle, physical activity level, and the dietary habits of the population in these very diverse countries. We can not simply say that heart disease is caused by fat consumption.

The famous *Seven Countries Study* was officially launched in 1958. Ancel Keys and his colleagues studied the relationship between diet, lifestyle and cardiovascular disease. The participating countries were *Greece, Italy, Yugoslavia, Netherlands, Finland, Japan* and the *United States*. The major finding of the study was that high cholesterol levels are associated with a high risk of heart disease mortality. In countries where people had high cholesterol, heart attacks were common; in countries where people had low cholesterol, heart attacks were rare. However, within individual countries major discrepancies

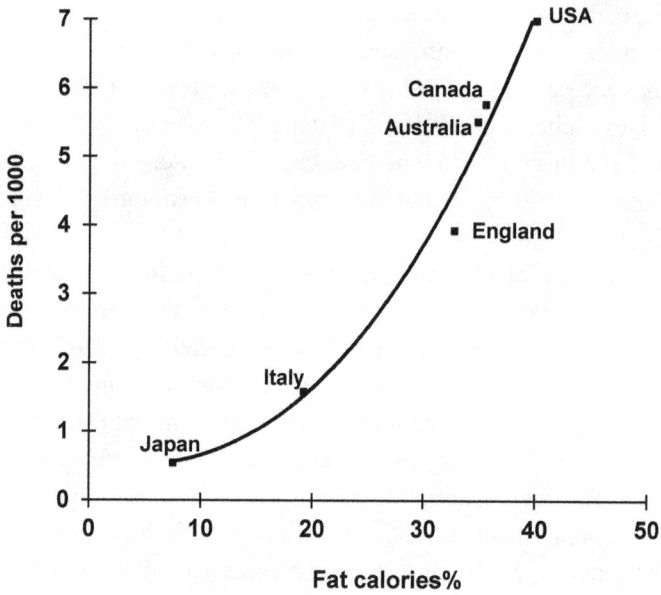

Figure 19.1. Ancel Keys' chart based on 6 countries

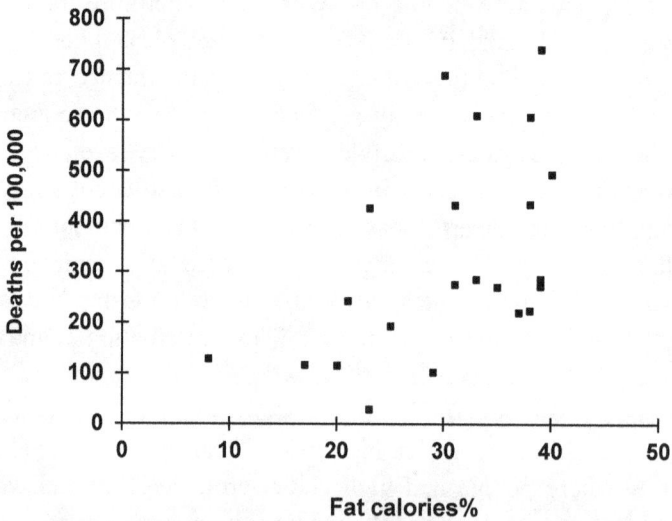

Figure 19.2. Chart based on the available 22 countries

were found. For example, in *North Karelia*, Finland, five times more people died from heart attack than those living in Turku, although blood cholesterol levels were the same. Those who lived on the Greek island *Corfu* had slightly lower cholesterol than those who lived on *Crete*, but had five times more heart attacks. In *Crevalcore*, Italy, the number of heart disease deaths was 2.5 times greater than in *Montegiorgio*, Italy, despite the fact that blood cholesterol levels were the same.

Although the cholesterol hysteria was synonymous with the name of *Ancel Keys*, even Keys himself wasn't even sure that dietary cholesterol raises blood cholesterol levels and causes heart disease. In a 1955 article, published in *The Journal of Nutrition*, he said: "Serum cholesterol level is essentially independent of the cholesterol intake".[69] Even decades later, in 1991, Ancel Keys was still a big-time skeptic of his own theory: "Adding cholesterol to a cholesterol free diet raises the blood levels in humans, but when added to an unrestricted diet, it has a minimal effect".[70]

THE DIET-HEART HYPOTHESIS

The *diet-heart hypothesis* is considered by the mainstream medicine as a proven fact rather than just a theory. The hypothesis says that dietary fat raises blood cholesterol and therefore increases the risk of coronary heart disease. Although there are some elements of truth in the second part of the hypothesis, ie. high LDL levels may increase the risk of cardiovascular disease, the first part of the hypothesis has never been proven. Even *Ancel Keys* admitted the fact that dietary fat intake does NOT raise blood cholesterol.

The *Framingham Heart Study* (FHS) is one of the most frequently cited studies in the medical literature. It was a project of the *National Heart, Lung, and Blood Institute*. The main objective of the study was to identify the major risk factors for cardiovascular disease. The first phase began in 1948 with the participation of 5,209 adult subjects from Framingham Massachusetts. Running for more than half a century, the FHS had become a long-term, multigenerational study. In addition to the original participants, their children and even their grandchildren, have been involved as well. Framingham was among the first studies identifying smoking, high blood pressure, obesity, and physical inactivity as the major risk factors for coronary heart disease. The Framingham Heart Study also proved that there is no relationship between fat consumption and blood cholesterol levels.[71] This important discovery however, didn't receive much media attention.

The *Honolulu Heart Study* was conducted in Hawaii with the participation of men of Japanese ancestry. During a period of 6 years, 7,705 healthy men were followed to determine if they developed coronary heart disease. Over the course of the whole study, in total, 294 of the participants had heart disease. Researchers compared dietary habits, including cholesterol intake, between those two groups of subjects who remained healthy and those who developed or died from heart disease. Surprisingly, those who had heart attacks or died of coronary heart disease had slightly lower cholesterol intake than the healthy subjects (521 mg vs. 549 mg).[72]

We have previously mentioned that in the Western countries, a large number of clinical trials is founded by the pharmaceutical industry. Such biased studies don't really provide strong scientific evidence. As a comparison, let's take a closer look at a study that was conducted in two countries where the Big Pharma had virtually zero influence. In 1977, right in the middle of the communist era and the cold war, a paper was published in *The American Journal of Clinical Nutrition*. A portion of the cited study was done in *Sofia, Bulgaria*, and another portion in *Prague, Czechoslovakia*. Researchers were studying how egg consumption influences blood cholesterol levels. Eggs are frequently used in clinical trials to evaluate the health effects of cholesterol intake, because eggs contain a relatively large amount of cholesterol, approximately 250 mg / 100 grams. The results from *Prague* and *Sofia* showed that adding two eggs to their daily diet didn't change the subjects' blood cholesterol level after a period of one week.[73] Both experiments confirmed that dietary cholesterol has no effect on blood cholesterol.

European researchers have proven that eating two eggs a day does not influence blood cholesterol levels at all. Let's see what happens if we eat not just two eggs, but much more than that. An article was published in *The New England Journal of Medicine* back in 1991. An 88 year-old man, who lived in a retirement home ate 25 eggs every single day the for last 15 years.[74] He always had soft boiled eggs and ate them throughout the day. Despite the excessive cholesterol intake, the old man maintained a normal blood cholesterol level. The consumption of 20 to 30 eggs a day was verified by the author of the article; the employees of the retirement home confirmed the daily delivery of approximately two dozen eggs.

SUMMARY

Cholesterol is often confused with the *low-density lipoproteins* (LDL) that are frequently referred to as the "bad cholesterol". Cholesterol *by itself* is absolutely harmless and is present in almost every single cell of our body as a building block of the cell membrane. Cholesterol is also an important component of bile and is the raw material of vitamin D and various hormones. Literally, there is no life without cholesterol. Every single day our body synthesizes approximately 700 milligrams of cholesterol. Dietary fat and cholesterol intake and blood cholesterol levels are virtually independent of each other. The more cholesterol you eat, the less cholesterol your body has to produce. On the other hand, if you are on a low cholesterol diet, your body has to make more cholesterol than you normally would. As we saw from this chapter, for most people, being on a cholesterol free diet is useless.

20

THE BIG WHITE KILLER

DISEASES OF CIVILIZATION

Traditionally, fat tissue was viewed merely as the long-term energy depot of the body to store excess calories. However, the results of the latest research show that besides the energy storage function, fat tissue is a highly active metabolic and endocrine organ as well. Fat cells produce hormones and *cytokines* that serve as signaling molecules. Some of these cytokines have an adverse effect on our health. They keep the body in a state of a continuous, *low-grade inflammation.* Most of the diseases of our modern-day lifestyle such as obesity, type-2 diabetes, cardiovascular disease, stroke, arthritis and cancer are associated with a continuous, low-grade inflammation. Since refined carbohydrates have the most fattening effect of all nutrients, they are closely linked to our diseases of civilization.

Cancer, diabetes and cardiovascular disease were still very rare in the beginning of the 20th century. For example, in his 1921 medical textbook, *William Osler* – often referred to as "the father of modern medicine" – mentioned that among the 27,618 patients of the *Johns Hopkins Hospital,* there were only 276 cases of diabetes.[75] This is only one percent, just a small fraction of today's rates. During the last one hundred years, the prevalence of obesity and diabetes has been steadily increasing alongside our sugar consumption. In the United States, between 1990 and 2015, the prevalence rate of diabetes increased from 5.3% to 8.4%. The statistics are alarming: the number of diabetic people is 8 times higher than a hundred years earlier. The diabetes epidemic is not limited only to America or to the Western world. The rates are increasing rapidly in developing countries as well. See Figure 20.1.

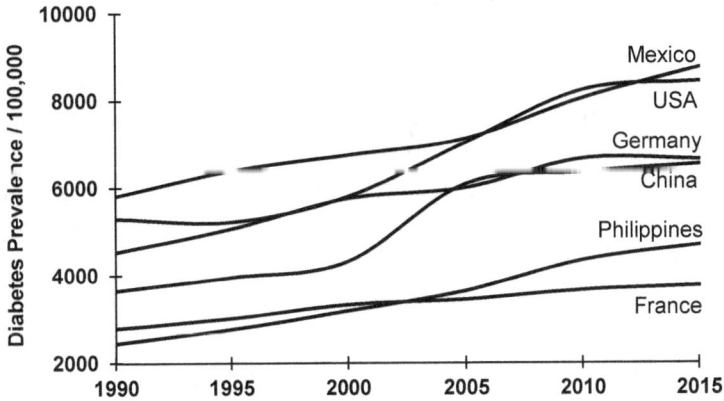

Figure 20.1. Increasing rates of diabetes worldwide

THE FATTENING CARBOHYDRATES

The fattening effect of refined carbohydrates has been well known since the early 19th century. 200 years ago, French polymath, *Brillat-Savarin* warned us that carbohydrates in both foods and beverages cause obesity. Until the 1960s, there was still a consensus among leading scientists about the fattening effect of carbohydrates. In 1963, *Dr. Passmore* and *Dr. Swindells* started their article in the *British Journal of Nutrition* with the following statement[39]: "Every woman knows that carbohydrate is fattening: this is a piece of common knowledge, which few nutritionists would dispute."

Since the 1960s however, with the outbreak of the great heart disease epidemic, public policies drastically changed towards carbohydrate consumption. While dietary fat had suddenly become one of the major risk factors for coronary heart disease, the well-known fattening effects of carbohydrates just got ignored. All kinds of carbohydrate foods were acceptable as long as they were cholesterol free. The 1991 pamphlet of the *American Heart Association* called the following foods healthy: white bread, hard candy, gum drops, sugar, syrup, honey, jam, jelly, marmalade, fruit punches and carbonated soft drinks. Even up to 12 ounces (0.36 liters) of beer (!) was on the list of the recommended healthy foods. A perfect recipe for disaster. It was no wonder the introduction of the new U.S.

dietary guidelines coincided with the beginning of the greatest obesity epidemic in human history.

Fats have been playing an important role in our diet since the dawn of the civilization. In contrast, *refined sugar* doesn't occur naturally; originally it wasn't part of our diet. It has only been mass produced since the 19th century. As our sugar consumption gradually increased over the course of the last two centuries, so did the prevalence rates of obesity, diabetes, cancer and cardiovascular disease. Interestingly, during World War I and World War II, when people faced food shortage and rationing, civilization diseases temporarily receded. When the war was over, the rates climbed even higher than before.

Among people who lived in a natural environment and ate natural food (such as the Native Americans, Pacific Islanders and African tribal communities) obesity, coronary heart disease, cancer and diabetes were virtually non-existent until the end of the 19th century. For example, the world famous missionary doctor *Albert Schweitzer* was astonished to encounter no cases of cancer upon his arrival in Gabon in 1913. Several years after the introduction of European processed foods however, cancer appeared among the locals who replaced their traditional diet with Western food.

SUGAR MAFIA

The United States Senate's *Select Committee on Nutrition and Human Needs* published a pamphlet back in 1977, entitled *Dietary Goals for the United States*. Health authorities told people to increase their carbohydrate consumption to 55-60 percent of their total energy intake and reduce fat consumption from approximately 40 to 30 percent. Unfortunately, Americans took this BAD advice. The introduction of the new dietary guidelines coincided with the beginning of the largest obesity epidemic in human history. Let's take a closer look what caused the derailment of scientific research for half a century. Was it just an accident or were there some hidden forces diverting research into a wrong direction?

The *Sugar Research Foundation* was founded by the members of the U.S. sugar industry in 1943. Their role was funding and sponsoring scientific research related to sugar and its by-products. In other words, they financed researchers likely to produce "scientific evidence" that supported the health benefits of sugar consumption and suppressed those results that associate sugar with adverse health effects. I'd like to point out that the *Sugar Research Foundation* played a similar role as the *Council for Tobacco Research* in the funding of tobacco-related research programs. In 1965, the *Sugar Research Foundation* secretly funded a study that was published in the *New England Journal of Medicine*. The paper discounted the evidence that sugar consumption is associated with coronary heart disease.[76] The funding role of the Sugar Research Foundation was not disclosed.

Based on internal documents from the sugar industry, a study called *Project 259* ran from 1967 to 1971. Researchers found that sugar intake is associated with a higher risk for coronary heart disease than starch consumption is. The other important finding of the experiment was that sugar is a potential carcinogen[76] (a cancer-causing substance). The *Sugar Research Foundation* wasn't happy with the outcome at all. They simply terminated *Project 259* without publishing the results. In 2016, the *Sugar Association*, the former *Sugar Research Foundation*, issued a press release criticizing a study published in the prestigious medical journal called *Cancer Research*. The authors of the condemned paper proved that high sugar consumption has a significant impact on the development of breast cancer.[77] Researchers found that Western style diets not only stimulate tumor growth but also accelerate cancer metastasis.

The fattening effect of sugar-sweetened beverages is a well-known fact. From time to time we come across studies however, showing "scientific evidence" that sugary drinks are not linked to obesity. Researchers compared industry-funded studies to those ones that had no conflict of interest. It turned out that studies funded by the sugar industry are 5 times more likely to present a conclusion that there is no association between sugar consumption and obesity.[78]

These examples were meant to illustrate the fact that the food industry, just like Big Pharma had corrupted scientific research. Because of an obvious conflict of interest, scientific evidence based on industry sponsored studies should be discredited.

21

HEART MAFIA

THE MULTI-BILLION DOLLAR BUSINESS

Coronary heart disease is the number one cause of death in the U.S. Cardiovascular disease not only claims more lives than any of the greatest wars did in the history of the United States, but it also puts an enormous financial burden on society. Based on the *American Heart Association's* 2016 statistics, cardiovascular disease costs America $555 billion.

Angioplasty is the most frequently performed surgical procedure done by cardiologists. Angioplasty is not a recent invention, it has been around for a while. It was invented in 1964 by *Charles Dotter*, who was later also nominated for the Nobel Prize. Angioplasty is a therapeutic procedure to treat the narrowed coronary arteries of the heart. The intervention involves guiding a catheter with a deflated balloon to the affected region of the body. A wire is passed through the narrowing and the balloon is inflated by using water. The balloon forces the expansion of the blood vessel. After removing the balloon, the intervention allows for improved blood flow (see Figure 21.1). A stent (a metal or plastic tubing to reinforce the vessel) may or may not also be placed. The whole procedure typically takes from 30 to 60 minutes. In case of a heart attack, angioplasty is literally a life-saver. The same is not true when angioplasty is done to open up narrowed arteries that aren't causing any problems. Many cardiologists think that the majority of these procedures are unnecessary. In the case of stable angina, angioplasty doesn't prolong life or prevent future heart attacks. Readers may ask the question: why are all these unnecessary procedures performed on a regular basis? The answer is very simple. Angioplasty surgery is a multi-billion dollar business. Over half a million patients are going through angioplasty in the

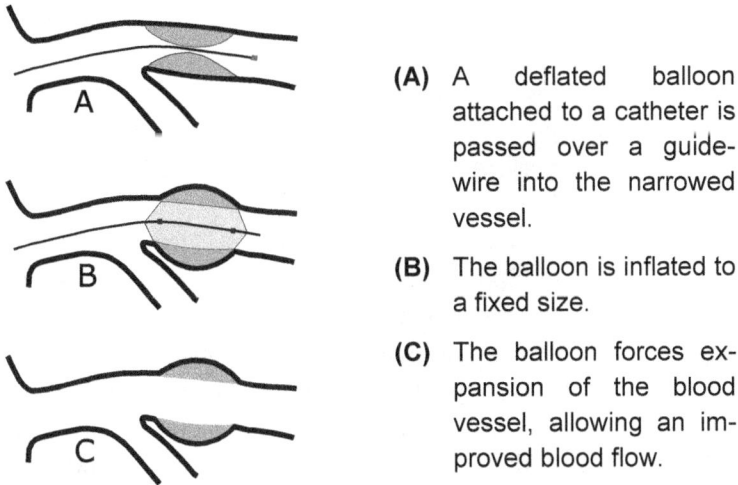

(A) A deflated balloon attached to a catheter is passed over a guide-wire into the narrowed vessel.

(B) The balloon is inflated to a fixed size.

(C) The balloon forces expansion of the blood vessel, allowing an improved blood flow.

Figure 21.1. Balloon angioplasty

United States with an average cost of $28,200, totaling more than 14 billion dollars each year.

I'd like to emphasize that this chapter of the book applies to *stable angina* only; in case of acute coronary syndrome angioplasty may be a life-saving intervention. Stable angina is chest pain or discomfort caused by the obstruction of a coronary artery. Symptoms most often occur during physical activity or emotional stress. Symptoms diminish several minutes after physical activities stop and recur when activities resume. The procedure of angioplasty does not offer a real solution to the problem, as it just suppresses the symptoms without treating the underlying cause of the disease. Angina is ultimately caused by atherosclerosis, a condition involving the obstruction of the arteries due to fatty deposits on the arterial walls. Atherosclerosis is a metabolic disorder that can not be treated by surgical procedures. Only radical changes implemented in the individual's lifestyle such as adopting a healthy diet, a physically active lifestyle, and reducing stress levels can eliminate those factors causing the disease.

EVIDENCE AGAINST ANGIOPLASTY

A study was published in the prestigious British medical journal *The Lancet*.[79] In the ORBITA study, 230 patients with severe ischemic symptoms ($\geq$70% single-vessel stenoses) were enrolled. Half of the subjects went through an angioplasty, while the other half had just a *placebo*, a fake surgery. After the procedure, patients received a 6-week treatment and their physical performance was evaluated. The physical strength was measured by the length of time the subjects were able to exercise. Surprisingly in both groups, among those who underwent the real surgery and those who had just a placebo surgery, the physical performance improved. There was just a minor difference between the two groups. In other words, the study has proved that angioplasty performed on patients with stable angina is useless.

A larger-scale study was performed in the United States and Canada with the participation of 2,287 subjects who suffered from significant coronary artery disease.[80] Half of the patients underwent angioplasty, while the other half just received a regular medical treatment. During the period of the next 2.5 to 7 years, the participants were monitored; and the occurrence of deaths and myocardial infarction (heart attack) was analyzed. Researchers found no difference between the number of heart attacks, strokes or deaths between the two groups. Angioplasty didn't reduce the risk of future cardiac events.

These results were confirmed by a third study with 5,286 participants. In those patients with stable coronary artery disease who underwent angioplasty, the procedure did not reduce the risk of future heart attacks or death.[81]

The uselessness of angioplasty in cases of *stable angina* may seem a little bit off-topic. My intention was expressing my growing concern that today's Western medicine heavily relying on drugs and unnecessary surgical procedures got hijacked by the healthcare mafia.

PART

FOUR

DR. TOROK'S ULTIMATE FOOD GUIDE

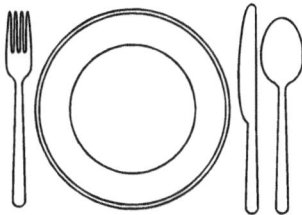

22

GLYCEMIC INDEX CONTROVERSIES

THE FATTENING EFFECT OF CARBOHYDRATES

We read in *The Formula for Weight Loss* chapter that foods rich in easily digestible carbohydrates, especially in sugar and starch, produce *hyperinsulinemia*, a condition with higher than normal blood insulin levels. Insulin diverts calories into fat cells, instead of using up the energy in lean tissues. That's why insulin has to be viewed as the main driving force behind obesity. In order to minimize those sudden blood glucose and insulin spikes following food intake, you should avoid foods rich in refined carbohydrates.

In addition to calories, there are several other indicators that can be used to evaluate the various properties of foods. These parameters cannot be ignored, since they are almost as important as the energy content of foods themselves. The concept of *glycemic index* was developed by Dr. David Jenkins at the University of Toronto in 1981. The theory that revolutionized the diet industry was originally meant for diabetic patients to manage their carbohydrate load.

Glycemic index (GI) is one of the most widely-used concepts in nutrition science, although it is very often misquoted and misunderstood. The glycemic index is a ranking of carbohydrates on a scale from 0 to 100 according to their blood sugar raising properties after eating. That's basically what *glycemic index* is; nothing more, nothing less. *Glycemic index* does NOT qualify the food itself and especially does not measure the fattening effect of various food items. If all of these things weren't confusing enough, let's see how *glycemic index* is calculated. Subjects eat an experimental meal, containing 50 grams of carbohydrates. During the following two hours, several blood samples are taken to evaluate the increase in blood sugar levels. The glucose-raising effect of the food is calculated by the *incremental area under the curve* (AUC) method. The AUC values are then compared to a reference food, either glucose or white bread. The *glycemic index* of the test food is calculated by dividing the glucose AUC for the test food by the glucose AUC for the reference food, then multiplied by 100.

The use of *glycemic index* has several limitations. As mentioned earlier, GI does NOT qualify the food itself; it is limited to the food's carbohydrate portion only. The rest of the nutrients are simply ignored. Certain amino acids stimulate the release of insulin which is well known for its fattening effect. The other concern is that this method does not take into consideration the fact that dietary fats slow down glucose absorption rate. The fiber content of the food is ignored as well. Furthermore, the *glycemic index* doesn't even take into account the actual carbohydrate content of the food. The calculated glycemic index is determined by a preset amount of food containing 50 grams of carbohydrates. Although a fancy glycemic index table is an indispensable part of every stylish diet website, the method by itself has very limited practical use.

In 1997, the concept of *glycemic load* was invented by Harvard scientists as a quick fix for the shortfalls of the glycemic index. Glycemic load is the product of the carbohydrate content in a typical serving of food and the *glycemic index* of the food, then divided by 100. With the introduction of *glycemic load* we've got just one step closer to the truth. However, the whole concept is still outdated because all the non-carbohydrate nutrients are ignored, despite the fact that some of them have a significant impact on the absorption rate of carbohydrates.

Because insulin is the main driving force behind obesity, it would be more practical to measure blood insulin levels directly, instead of blood glucose levels. The *food insulin index* is calculated by the following formula: insulin response to test food divided by insulin response to reference food (glucose or white bread) then multiplied by 100. The *insulin index* is based on food samples with an energy content of 1000 kJ (240 kcal). With the invention of *food insulin index* scientists managed to overcome most of the limitations of *glycemic index*. Since the concept of *food insulin index* is still relatively new, it is less widely used than *glycemic index*. Table 22.1 on the next page shows the insulin index of a few food items. Column 2 lists the insulin index of foods and column 3 shows the weight of foods containing 1000 kJ (240 kcal) of energy. The lower the number in column 3, the higher the energy density of the food item. The table reveals a few important facts: whole grain products always have a significantly lower insulin index than the refined version of the same food (whole-wheat bread vs. white bread, brown rice vs. white rice). Skim milk raises insulin levels 2.5 times more than whole milk. Some sweets increase blood insulin even higher than pure sugar: with an insulin index of 117, Jellybeans are the marvel of modern-day junk food engineering!

If we are trying to evaluate the fattening effect of different foods, the *food insulin index* is the best of all existing methods previously discussed. In case the *insulin index* of a certain food is not available, using *glucose score* is the best choice. *Glucose score* is similar to *glycemic index*, however the quantity of the test and reference food is not based on 50 grams of carbohydrate content but on 1000 kJ of energy. *Glucose score* can be calculated from the glycemic index, energy and the carbohydrate content of the food.

Knowing the blood glucose and insulin raising properties of the foods we eat is indispensable. Besides, there are a few other things to which we need to pay attention. When reading *glycemic index / insulin index* tables, we need to take into consideration whether the data is based on raw or cooked food. Cooking increases the digestibility of foods. Raw or partially cooked foods affect blood glucose and insulin levels to a smaller extent than fully cooked meals. The ripeness of fruits greatly influences their digestibility. As starches are gradually converted into sugars during the ripening process, the glycemic index of the fruits significantly increases. The processing method of the food ingredients also has a great impact on their digestibility. Small particle sizes increase surface area and accelerate digestion. For example, fine flour has a significantly higher insulin raising effect than coarse floor.

Food item	Insulin index	240 kcal, grams
White bread	73	97
Whole-wheat bread	50	95
White rice, cooked	55	159
Brown rice, cooked	29	149
Apples	43	435
Bananas	59	279
Avocado	4	112
Oranges	44	625
Grapes	60	395
Coleslaw	20	252
Carrots	44	775
Peanuts	15	38
Eggs	23	160
Tuna, canned in water	26	239
White fish	43	333
Chicken, fried	19	94
Milk, whole	24	368
Milk, skim	60	690
Cheese, Cheddar	33	59
Butter	2	33
Olive oil	3	27
Mars bar	89	54
Jellybeans	117	88

Table 22.1. Insulin index and the weight of foods containing 240 kcal

We can conclude that the fattening effect of foods is closely related to their refined carbohydrate content and the degree of processing. Highly processed foods with concentrated carbohydrate content are the most fattening ones.

23

HOW TO READ FOOD LABELS

COW FIELD AND MARTIAN SECONDS

Do you know what's common about *cow field*, *Martian seconds* and
the food labels in the United States? Let me explain it for those who
haven't heard about it, *cow field* is a British unit of measurement,
equal to the amount of land that could produce enough grass to
support a cow. A Martian second is the length of a second on the
planet of Mars. Imagine how much confusion it would cause if train
schedules were posted in Martian hours and Martian minutes, or if
building lots were sold based on how many cows they can support?
The food labeling system in the United States is not less confusing
than the use of *cow field* or *Martian seconds*. Take a look at *Figure
23.1* that shows a sample U.S. food label. What do you think the total
carbohydrate content of that particular food is? At first look we may
think the food contains 13% of carbohydrates, because that's the
number you can read on the label. A HUGE **FAT** LIE! The fact of
the matter is, the actual carbohydrate content is 100 x 37/55 = 67%.
Food labels are designed that way on purpose. Food manufacturers
don't want the average consumers to know exactly what's in the food
they eat. Unfortunately, such purposely misleading labeling practice
is absolutely legal in the US and Canada. Here comes the explanation: the percentage figures on labels do not display the actual nutrient content of the food; they are based on "daily values" instead. The
only thing labels show is the percentage of one serving's nutrient
content compared to the recommended daily intake. Since serving
sizes are arbitrary, the figures can be easily manipulated. Those who
want to know the exact nutrient content, need to use the following
formula:

100 x weight of the nutrient in grams / serving size in grams

For example:

The *real* fiber content from the sample label is 7% (100 x 4 / 55).

A free food label nutrient calculator is available on the author's website. Scan the code on the right with your device.

Nutrition Facts

8 servings per container

Serving size   2/3 cup (55g)

Amount per serving

Calories   **230**

	% Daily Value*
Total Fat 8g	**10%**
Saturated Fat 1g	**5%**
Trans Fat 0g	
Cholesterol 0mg	**0%**
Sodium 160mg	**7%**
Total Carbohydrate 37g	**13%**
Dietary Fiber 4g	**14%**
Total Sugars 12g	
Includes 10g Added Sugars	**20%**
Protein 3g	
Vitamin D2mcg10%	
Calcium 260mg	20%
Iron 8 mg	45%
Potassium 235mg 6%	

* The % Daily Value (DV) tells you how much a nutrient in a serving of food contributes to a daily diet. 2,000 calories a day is used for general nutrition advice.

Figure 23.1. Nutrition Facts label from the United States, as of 2016

In our example, the actual carbohydrate content is 5 times higher and the fiber content is just half of the amount that the label suggests. Doesn't it sound like food manufacturers are simply cheating on their food labels?

In countries where the food lobby is less influential, for example in the EU, this kind of purposeful misinformation is not allowed. In the EU, every food label has to display the *actual* energy and nutrient content on a percentage basis. By doing that, the nutrient content of different food items can be easily compared, even by non-experts. Junk food companies don't need well-informed consumers. Remember the old Rockefeller saying: "I don't want a nation of thinkers".

LITTLE LIES

Food labels contain tons of false statements. The term *sugar free* is one of those. If a food is sold as *sugar free* it doesn't necessarily mean that there is zero sugar in it, as we would naturally think. As per the FDA's *Food Labeling Guide*, *sugar free* foods may contain up to 0.5 grams of sugar *per serving*.

Trans fats are created from unsaturated fatty acids by chemical treatment. Since they don't occur naturally, we should completely eliminate them from our diet. From the manufacturers' point of view, labeling a food as a "zero trans fat" product is a good selling feature. Are these food items really trans fat free? Not necessarily. FDA regulations allow companies to label a product as "zero trans fat" if it contains no more than 0.5 grams of trans fat *per serving*.

On food labels we often come across the word "natural". Does it mean that the product contains no artificial ingredients? Not at all. The term "natural" is actually not regulated by FDA. So-called "natural" foods may contain high-fructose corn syrup (corn is natural after all) or even GMO products. In the United States, there were several court cases where individuals sued companies who were claiming the right to continue labeling such food items as "natural". Food manufacturers often use *"natural flavors"*. Although the raw materials of these ingredients originally come from natural sources, they still contain large amounts of solvents, preservatives and other chemicals.

Junk food manufacturers often make claims like "made with real fruit" when selling their products loaded with high-fructose corn syrup, preservatives, artificial flavors, coloring and other chemicals. Such foods don't contain much fruit, if they have real fruit at all. Companies are not required by law to disclose the fruit content of their products. In a federal court in California *Kellogg* was sued for false advertising on their *Super Mario* fruit snacks, claiming it was "made with real fruit". Instead of real fruit, the product was composed of sugar, corn syrup, apple puree concentrate, artificial flavors, coloring and other additives.

The fattening effect of sugars is a well-known fact. Since sugars are not a good selling feature on food labels, manufacturers very often disguise sugar under different names. Those guys are very creative. Even if the ingredient's name on the label does not contain the word *sugar*, the chemical name of that particular sugar may be used, such as glucose, dextrose, fructose, lactose, maltose, sucrose, disaccharides or monosaccharides. Frequently, high sugar content ingredients are listed on food labels without using the word *sugar*, for example: syrup, nectar, honey, caramel or molasses.

Food manufacturers can purchase a heart-check food certification from the *American Heart Association*. For paying an annual fee of $3,000 to $6,000 per item, the product is entitled to the famous heart check logo. I hope you don't think you will live to be a hundred, never have a heart attack, and stay healthy forever simply by eating food recommended by the American Heart Association. To get a food approved, the manufacturer has to meet just the bare minimum. Salt, fat and cholesterol content is limited (plant foods don't contain cholesterol anyways). These rules are very vague. Although added sugar is limited to 5 grams per serving for snack foods, serving sizes are not determined. Naturally occurring sugars do not count toward this limit. In other words, there is no upper limit on total sugar content.

24

BEWARE OF SUGAR

THE DANGERS OF SUGAR CONSUMPTION

The fattening effect of refined carbohydrates is a proven scientific fact that has been known for 200 years. Traditionally, fat tissue was viewed merely as a long-term storage media for excess calories. However, the results of the latest research show that besides its storage function, fat tissue is a highly active metabolic and endocrine organ as well. In *The Big White Killer* chapter we saw that fat cells produce hormones and cytokines that serve as signaling molecules. Some of these cytokines have an adverse health effect. They keep the body in the state of a continuous, low-grade inflammation. Most of the diseases of our modern-day lifestyle such as obesity, type-2 diabetes, cardiovascular disease, stroke, arthritis and cancer are associated with a continuous, low-grade inflammation. Decades, or many years of constant exposure to a state of a continuous inflammation predispose us to such diseases.

Until the 1960s, there was still a consensus among leading scientists about the fattening effect of refined carbohydrates. In the *Fattening Carbohydrates* chapter, we discussed that at the beginning of the great heart disease epidemic, mainstream scientists and health authorities changed their minds and dietary fat had suddenly become one of the major risk factors for coronary heart disease and obesity. Although such claims cannot really be supported with solid scientific evidence, the *diet-heart hypothesis* became the most widely accepted view held by mainstream scientists. In the infamous 1977 publication entitled *Dietary Goals for the United States*, US health authorities told citizens that they could improve their health by reducing the fat in their diets and increasing their carbohydrate consumption. Unfortunately, people took the bad advice and did exactly what they were told to do: reduced their fat intake and increased carbohydrate consumption. It is no wonder that the new dietary guidelines coincided with the beginning of the largest obesity epidemic in human history.

If we look back in history a little bit earlier, we will see that a couple of centuries ago, before its mass production, sugar was only available to the elite classes who could afford it. As production increased and prices dropped, the precious commodity became an everyday item. During the past two hundred years, the average American's sugar intake rose nine fold. As sugar production gradually went up during the last two centuries, the prevalence rate of civilization diseases such as cancer, heart disease, stroke and type-2 diabetes increased parallelly with our sugar consumption.

Many scientists agree that *refined* sugar causes addiction. In other words, most of us are sugar addicts. Our addiction starts in early childhood. Baby formulas and canned baby foods contain way more sugar than necessary. Manufacturers overdose sugar in children's food on purpose. At a very early age, children become trained to love super-sweet flavors. Food companies are doing this on purpose: they raise a new generation of sugar addicts.

What is the ideal solution to the problem of sugar addiction? Given the addictive nature of refined sugar, there is only one fix that works in the long run: eliminating *refined* sugar from our *everyday* diet; this should be one of our top priorities. Foods with naturally occurring *unrefined* carbohydrates such as cereals, fruits and vegetables have been part of our diet since ancient times. However, the *concentrated* amounts of refined carbohydrates from highly processed food definitely make us obese and sick in the long run. All kinds of engineered food needs to be completely avoided. Once you get rid of the fast-digestible carbohydrates in your diet, you will prevent high insulin peaks following carbohydrate consumption. By lowering insulin levels, the calories will be burned in lean tissues instead of storing the excess energy in fat cells. By limiting the activity level of adipocytes (fat cells), the production of inflammation-causing cytokines will significantly decrease. As we have seen earlier, most of our modern-day civilization diseases are linked to a continuous low-grade inflammation in our body. By preventing inflammation, you will greatly reduce the risk for many modern-day diseases that are virtually non-existent in primitive societies such as heart disease, stroke, type-2 diabetes, cancer and many others.

There are two things I'd like to emphasize here. First, you don't need to give up eating sugar completely. When you reach your target body weight, you can still have some dessert on special occasions, once in a while; let's say one serving a week. Second, other forms of sugar, naturally occurring in fruits can be eaten even more frequently.

ARE YOU A SUGAR ADDICT?

There is a good chance that you are. Take your time, and calculate the amount of sugar you consume added to your food and beverages during an average day. Read food labels thoroughly. Be careful, food companies cheat on food labeling. In the previous chapter (*How to Read Food Labels*), I gave a practical guide on how to read food labels. You will be shocked by how much *unnecessary* sugar you eat every single day. An average American consumes 76 pounds of sugar annually. Imagine that you pile up 19 four-pound sugar bags on the shelves of your pantry. Sugar is added to virtually every single food item. Besides those foods where sugar is obviously present such as in pops, ice cream, snacks, cookies, desserts, chocolate or candies, sugar is added in smaller quantities to other food items where you wouldn't even expect. For example, many meat products contain added sugar. Since "healthy" foods are low in fat, in order to make them taste just a little bit better than saw dust, fats are replaced with sugar, salt and artificial flavors. Sugar is also added to bakery products, breakfast cereals, dairy products, salads and dressings. The vast majority of prepackaged foods contains a considerable amount of refined carbohydrate.

Scientists at Princeton University have proven that sugar, similarly to drugs, causes addiction.[82] Sugar addiction is associated with the use of the same brain pathways that are activated by addictive drugs. Four components of drug addiction are also present in the case of sugar addiction. The first component is *bingeing,* which means the intake of large amounts of food. *Withdrawal* is the second. Similarly to opiates, when the abused substance is no longer available, symptoms include anxiety and behavioral depression. The third component is *craving*, which is defined as increased efforts to obtain the substance being abused. Researchers identified the fourth component of addiction as well: *cross-sensitization*. Being sensitized to one drug may show increased intake of a different drug.

THE CRIME OF HIGH-FRUCTOSE CORN SYRUP

Glucose and *fructose* are the most common sugars in our diet. The absorbed glucose from the digested food is transported by the blood to the cells of our body. Starch from our food is broken down into small glucose units and then is taken up by the blood stream. The ingestion of both glucose and starches causes a significant increase in blood sugar level. *Fructose* is different however, it doesn't follow the same metabolic pathway. *Fructose* has just a minimal effect on blood sugar. That's why *fructose* is traditionally used in diabetic foods.

The results of latest research however, show that *fructose* is not as harmless as it seems. Excessive fructose consumption leads to serious health conditions. Most cells of the body have limited fructose (GLUT-5) transporters. Since the majority of cells are unable to uptake fructose, most of it will end up in the liver. Fructose stimulates building up fat deposits in the liver, ultimately leading to a serious health condition known as *nonalcoholic-fatty liver disease*. In addition to these adverse health effects, fructose can also be linked to the development of dyslipidemia and insulin resistance.

Another problem is that since fructose does not raise blood sugar levels, it doesn't give the signal to your brain that "it was enough". Remember when you were a child, eating sugar before your meal would "spoil your dinner" by suppressing your appetite. Fructose works differently than glucose, because it doesn't affect *ghrelin*, the major appetite-stimulating hormone. If you drink a large Coke with your meal at McDonalds, does the 320-calorie supersized fructose drink satisfy your appetite? Not at all. It will make you even hungrier.

Between 1970 and 2000, the per capita consumption of high-fructose corn syrup in the United States went up from 0.4 grams per day to 45.6 grams. This is a 114-time increase. Why did fructose become so popular? There are two good reasons. First, it has the most intensely sweet taste of all sugars. Since early childhood, we were programmed to love super-sweet flavors. Second, cultivating genetically modified corn is the cheapest way to mass produce sugar.

ARTIFICIAL SWEETENERS

The evidence proving the harmful effects of refined sugar is overwhelming. Dieters often use non-caloric sweeteners as a "healthy" alternative to fattening sugars. After all, these sweeteners contain zero calories. We may ask the question: Is replacing sugar with artificial sweeteners a good idea? The answer is definitely no. Artificial sweeteners cause even more trouble than sugar itself.

From time to time, we come across news that replacing sugar-sweetened beverages with diet sodas is a healthy choice and an efficient way to combat obesity. Clinical trials are often cited presenting the "scientific evidence" of the positive health effects of non-caloric sweeteners. Those studies aren't even worth the paper they are written on. As you may suspect, such experiments are typically sponsored by the big food companies. The British newspaper *The Independent*, mentioned a study claiming that diet drinks are even better than water at helping people lose weight.[83] The study was supported by a research institute, ILSI Europe, which is funded by its member companies such as Coca Cola or PepsiCo. In the case of such industry-supported studies, the outcome of the trial is already known even before the experiments started.

There are several adverse health effects associated with artificial sweeteners. Although they don't affect blood sugar levels directly, non-caloric sweeteners lower the body's insulin sensitivity. As a result of an impaired insulin sensitivity, the pancreas has to produce more insulin; this hormone is the main regulator of our body weight. In the process of diverting calories into fat deposits, blood insulin levels are even more important than blood glucose levels.

A 24-week trial was done with the participation of 89 overweight and obese women.[84] One group of the women had 5 diabetic beverages a week after their lunch, the other group drank water. Both groups were on a calorie-restricted diet. After 24 weeks, the water group achieved a 1.2 kg more weight reduction on average. The decrease in insulin levels was found to be 1.1 mU/L higher in the water group then in the diabetic beverage group. These numbers prove that artificial sweeteners cause insulin resistance and significantly increase the risk of obesity.

Another study found that in obese individuals, the intake of artificial sweeteners (sucralose), compared to water consumption[85] results in an 8% higher total insulin secretion.

Besides their adverse health effects, artificial sweeteners cause a probably even bigger problem: all sweeteners maintain cravings for super-sweet flavors. Since we are addicted to the sweet taste, non-caloric sweeteners when added to other meals, increase the amount of food we consume. So the net balance is definitely weight gain instead of weight loss.

Although commercially available sweeteners are approved by health authorities, their long-term health effect is still unknown. According to the *National Cancer Institute*, artificial sweeteners caused cancer in laboratory animals. To evaluate the long-term health effects on humans, unbiased, independent studies are necessary.

PRACTICAL ADVICE

By taking the advantage of sugar's addictive nature and in order to increase their sales figures, food manufacturers, add sugar to virtually every single food item. Sugar may be added even to products that you would never even suspect. For example, meat products, bread or even vinegar can contain a generous amount of sugar. As a general rule, avoid all foods with added sugar. Food labels should be always carefully studied.

The French polymath, *Brillat-Savarin* 200 years ago warned us that carbohydrates in beverages are as fattening as those in foods. Since then, the fattening effect of carbohydrates in liquids is well known, but we don't pay enough attention to that fact. In order to achieve a substantial amount of weight loss, we should completely avoid ALL types: pops, fruit juices, punches, beers, smoothies, flavored milks and flavored yogurt drinks.

We have previously mentioned that all foods with added sugar should be eliminated. What about those food items that have a very intense sweet taste but don't contain any added sugar? A very good question. Remember, we are all sugar addicts. A sweet taste is the main selling feature of almost every single food. Manufacturers don't lack creativity. To produce a "zero added sugar" product, sometimes they use naturally occurring ingredients with an elevated sugar content such as honey, fruit concentrates or syrups. Regardless of where the sugar comes from, these foods are equally bad.

Brown sugar is often marketed as a healthy alternative to white sugar. As a matter of fact, the only difference between the two types is that brown sugar contains some residual molasses from the manufacturing process. Sometimes manufacturers just simply add some brown stuff to refined white sugar. I regret to say that brown sugar is just as bad as white sugar.

Honey is all natural. It is loaded with valuable micronutrients and antioxidants. Honey has a remarkable anti-inflammatory and antibiotic effect. There is one thing however, that outweighs these great health benefits. Honey is composed of 82% sugar. Despite its essential nutrients, honey still has a significant fattening effect. The same principle applies to other naturally occurring syrups such as the famous Canadian maple syrup. Because of their high sugar content, all types of syrups should be avoided.

As a closing thought, I would say that if you manage to overcome your sugar addiction, half of the battle against obesity is already won.

25

WHEAT, THE CEREAL KILLER?

IS WHEAT REALLY BAD?

From time to time we come across articles claiming that wheat consumption is detrimental to our health. Some authors even call wheat the "silent killer", while others refer to it as the "cereal killer". Legends often have a basis of some truth. In my opinion, bakery products that we can find on the shelves of supermarkets today, deserve to be called the "silent killer". Typically, they are composed of highly refined carbohydrates; from a nutritional point of view nearly as bad as table sugar. However, because of the bad reputation of adulterated bread products it wouldn't be fair to condemn wheat itself. Since the beginning of our civilization, wheat has been our staple food. We definitely need to distinguish between *real bread* and its cheap imitation that is commercially available.

Today's bread, although it may look very similar, is definitely not the same as was in the days of our grandparents. Traditionally, bread was viewed as the staple food of humankind, it was also considered as the symbol of life. I regret to say this, but today's fake bread is no longer the symbol of life, but rather just another typical product of the junk food industry. Let's take a closer look at how our bread gets spoiled and what the main differences are between traditional bread and its modern-day counterfeit. In bread production, from the first step to the last, everything is done the just the wrong way, including:

- the use of modern wheat varieties
- the processing of the grain
- the removal of the fiber
- the bleaching of the flour
- the use of harmful additives

Each of these steps are the equivalent of mass murder. Our toxic food is the primary cause of the majority of modern-day civilization diseases, including cardiovascular disease, stroke, diabetes, cancer and many others.

THE GREEN REVOLUTION

The term *Green Revolution* refers to a worldwide agricultural revolution that took place from the 1950s to the 1970s. *Norman Borlaug*, who is called the "Father of the Green Revolution" received the Nobel Peace Prize in 1970. Borlaug was one of the chief scientists of the *Rockefeller Foundation*. The Foundation financially supported the modernization of many developing countries.

Typical of the Rockefellers, every time they expanded their business by taking over a big chunk of the economy, it was also construed as a great gesture of their generosity and philanthropy at the same time. In the early 20th century, the Rockefellers developed a monopoly of the oil industry and acquired business interests in the chemical industry as well. The real goal of the *Green Revolution* was to replace the nations' sustainable traditional agriculture with a new model, heavily reliant on the use of chemicals, pesticides, fertilizers and fossil fuels in order to generate billions of dollars of revenue for the Rockefeller empire. As a result of the Green Revolution, traditional crop varieties were replaced with the newly engineered ones that required large amounts of pesticides and fertilizers. There are two great wheat varieties that fell prey to the Green Revolution: *Emmer* and *Einkorn*. Both of them had been cultivated since ancient times. Compared to the modern varieties, they are rich in fiber, protein, vitamins and minerals. Foods made from these ancient wheats have a much lower glycemic index and insulin index, therefore consuming the same amount of calories has a significantly less harmful effect on weight compared to modern wheat varieties.

THE ASSASSINATION OF WHEAT

We saw that modern wheat varieties are significantly less nutritious than *Emmer* and *Einkorn*, which served as the staple food of mankind for millennia. However the worst part still has to come. During the milling process the germ and bran part of the grain are removed. What is left behind consists of mostly starch. The flour is deprived of its natural fiber content and a significant amount of protein, vitamins and minerals is lost as well. Without the protective effect of fiber, starch will be digested much faster, resulting in a blood glucose spike and an insulin rush following ingestion.

The horror story of wheat processing is not over yet. Traditionally, wheat was ground by millstones, producing a relatively coarse flour. These days however, by passing through modern milling equipment, the starch fraction of the wheat kernels is literally pulverized. Grinding cereals into dust-like small particles increases surface area and accelerates digestion. The processing method has a serious impact on both the glycemic index and insulin index of the food as well.

The adulteration process of flour is not complete yet. Now come the chemists. The aging of flour naturally takes months. That rarely happens today. As per the *North American Millers' Association*, in the bleaching process, flour is exposed to chlorine gas or *benzoyl peroxide* to speed up the aging process. By the way, chlorine gas was used as a chemical weapon in World War I. As for *benzoyl peroxide*, this chemical has been banned by the European Union in food products.

Since modern milling processes deprive flour of its valuable nutrients, it's time to add something to improve the nutritional value. During the enrichment process, a portion of the lost minerals and vitamins is replaced with artificial ones. This is the point, where the miller's story ends. The flour is packaged and shipped.

In bakeries, numerous additives, flavors and colorants are used to make the product more appealing to customers and to improve the workability of the dough. In addition to those chemicals, there is a hundred-percent natural ingredient that needs to be mentioned. It is sugar. You may be surprised, but sugar is widely used not only in sweet pastry products but in regular bread as well. Why? Because it makes bread tastier for many of us. Remember, we are all sugar addicts.

SUMMARY

We can conclude that traditionally baked bread made from the right ingredients should be a part of our healthy, everyday diet. Unfortunately, commercially produced bread doesn't meet these criteria. In order to make nutritious bread, we should follow the traditional way used by our ancestors. The first step is choosing the right grain. All the modern wheats result in a poor quality bread. The best wheat varieties are the ancient ones: *Einkorn* (Triticum monococcum) and *Emmer* (Triticum dicoccum). If these ones are not available, *Spelt* (Triticum spelta) can also be used as a substitute, although it is just half-way between the ancient and the modern varieties in its nutritional value. If none of these wheats are available, *rye* also makes a good quality bread, and barley is also a good choice. It has a very high fiber and protein content. *Hulled barley* contains the inedible hull portion of the grain; it is used as animal feed. *Dehulled barley* and *hulless barley* is for human consumption. Never use *pearl barley*. It is the junk food version of barley with the bran and germ removed.

The second step is making the right flour. Modern mills literally pulverize wheat kernels resulting in a high glycemic index product. The right flour is coarse-ground, because larger particles slow down the digestion process. The ideal flour has no additives at all and it can be easily produced even in your own kitchen. There are different tabletop sized mills available, and it is worth shopping for them on *Ebay*. Baking your own bread is much easier than you think. Even kids can make cookies. Making bread is much simpler than making cookies. Bread has only four ingredients: flour, yeast, water and salt. Bread can be baked in any oven. Homemade bread is not only healthier but also tastes much better than fake bread loaded with tons of chemicals.

Commercially produced breads and other bakery products have a serious negative impact on our health and should be avoided. Food manufacturers are very creative. From time to time they come up with new ideas like fortified bread or multi-grain bread. Sometimes they just put brown colorant into white flour to create the illusion of whole-wheat bread. These sales techniques are very deceptive, however they don't change the fact that commercially produced breads simply fall into the junk food category.

OAT CEREALS

Oat products are popular breakfast cereals. Oat contains *beta-glucan*, a plant polysaccharide that is resistant to digestion and decreases blood glucose and cholesterol levels. However, care needs to be taken in choosing commercially available oat products. Do your own homework and study labels carefully, because the best-selling oat cereals are high in sugar. Make your breakfast from scratch. Use whole grain rolled oats without any additives. Rolled oats are manufactured by steaming and flattening whole grain oats to form large flakes. They shouldn't have any other ingredients than oats.

Be extra careful, even if you come across "Heart healthy" breakfast cereals. Despite the famous checkmark logo of the *American Heart Association*, such products still may be loaded with tons of sugar, artificial flavors and colors. Breakfast cereals with added sugar are made for sugar addicts. The same thing applies to "healthy" granola bars and other cereal snacks.

CORN IS NOT GOOD FOR YOU

In many countries, corn is the main staple food of the whole population. It plays an even more important role than wheat or rice in the nutrition of people. The fact of the matter is, that corn has the lowest nutritional value and the worst fattening effect among all cereals. Corn is widely cultivated not because of its goodness but for economic reasons: it has a much higher yield per acre than any other cereal. Did you know that up to 92% of corn is genetically modified in the United States?[86] The yield per acre of genetically engineered corn is three times higher than of wheat.

Corn has been traditionally used for livestock fattening. Cattle, hogs and poultry are typically fattened by feeding corn. *Foie gras* is an expensive European gourmet food. Foie gras is the liver of an extremely fat duck or goose, which are fattened by force-feeding corn by using a feeding tube. As a result of excessive corn feeding, the liver of the animals enormously enlarges with massive amounts of fat deposits in their liver cells. The same condition in humans is called *nonalcoholic fatty liver disease*. The exact mechanism of corn's fattening effect is not entirely known. When comparing corn to whole wheat, there are substantial differences between the nutritional values of the two cereals. For example, corn has significantly less fiber than whole wheat does. Dietary fiber has a remarkable protective effect against a whole range of chronic diseases. In addition to the higher dietary fiber content, wheat also contains more protein compared to corn.

I'd like to emphasize that, nearly 100% of *non-organic* corn available in American supermarkets is genetically modified. The long-term health effect of GMO foods is still unknown. Although genetically modified foods are declared to be safe by health authorities, we shouldn't take it at face value.

26

THE STORY OF RICE

THE GREEN REVOLUTION, AGAIN

In the previous chapter, we saw how the ancient crop varieties fell prey to the Green Revolution. The ecologically sustainable agriculture in the developing countries was replaced with aggressive models heavily depending on the use of chemicals, pesticides, fertilizers and fossil fuel. The Green Revolution significantly reduced the agricultural biodiversity, as it relied on just a limited number of high-yield varieties of each crop. Rice is no exception. According to the *Rice Association*, more than 40,000 varieties of cultivated rice are known to exist. However, only a few modified rice variants are being used to grow for food. Since the early 2000s new, genetically modified rice varieties are being approved worldwide.

CHOOSING THE RIGHT RICE

Asian rice is the plant species most commonly referred to as rice. *Asian rice* can be put into two subcategories: the sticky, short-grained *japonica* and the nonsticky, long-grained *indica* rice. Besides *Asian rice* other cultivated rice species include *African rice* and *wild rice*.

Depending on the processing type, rice can be divided into two categories: *brown rice* and *white rice*. Brown rice is whole-grain rice with the inedible outer husk removed. All white rice starts out as brown rice. The milling process removes the husk, bran, and germ. As for the insulin index, there is a significant difference between various types of rice. When shopping for rice, special attention needs to be paid to select the right one. The insulin index of a good rice can be as low as just half of a bad quality variety. As a general rule of thumb, we should always go with brown rice. Since the bran component of white rice is already removed, the vast majority of its fiber content is also lost. Without the protective effect of dietary fiber, the carbohydrate content of food is absorbed at a higher speed, causing a sudden insulin spike after ingestion.

During the processing, when white rice is produced, it also loses many of its valuable vitamins, especially *vitamin B1*. Historically, in those developing countries where white rice was the staple food of the population, a medical condition called *beriberi*, caused by vitamin B1 deficiency, was more common.

Starches are long chain molecules built up from glucose units. The starch content of rice is present in two forms: amylose and amylopectin. Amylopectin has branched chains and it is relatively easy to digest. Amylose molecules have a straight shape and they are digested at a slower rate. Varieties with a higher amylose content have a significantly lower glycemic index and insulin index. These are the nonsticky, long-grained types. Considering all commercially available rice varieties, the unpolished, brown *doongara* and *basmati* rice are the healthiest choice. Brown *basmati* rice is usually available in larger supermarkets and Indian stores.

Many Asian recipes contain rice flour. The same principle applies here as in the case of wheat flour. The smaller the particle size, the faster the rate of digestion is, which is not good for your health. Therefore, foods containing whole grain rice are preferred to those made with rice flour.

Finally, another piece of practical advice. As a general rule applicable to every other plant-based food: don't overcook your meal, just cook it as much as necessary. Cooking makes the starch content of the food more easily digestible and therefore increases its glycemic index.

27

MAN'S BEST FRIEND

THE BENEFITS OF FIBER

"Man's best friend" is a common phrase about dogs, referring to their long-lasting companionship with humans. Although today most dogs are kept as pets, for thousands of years dogs protected humans and their belongings. Just as dogs have guarded us for millennia, so has dietary fiber protected our health since ancient times. Fiber also deserves the title *man's best friend*, at least from a nutritional point of view. Dietary fiber has numerous health benefits, including reducing the risk of developing some cancers, hyperlipidemia, hypertension, coronary heart disease, and type-2 diabetes. Dietary fibers slow down the absorption rate of carbohydrates and reduce the post-meal insulin responses. As a result of lower insulin levels, less energy will be deposited in fat cells. When comparing foods with similar carbohydrate content, the higher the fiber content, the lower the insulin index is. Table 27.1. shows the insulin index and fiber content of various food items (For example, compare *whole-wheat bread* to *white bread* or *brown rice* to *white rice*). Fibers also delay gastric emptying, which results in an extended feeling of fullness.

The *Dietary Guidelines for Americans* 2010 Edition recommends a daily fiber intake of 25 grams for women and 38 grams for men. Although these values fall within the norms of international recommendations, mainstream nutrition science seems to be grossly underestimating the adequate intake of dietary fiber. In order to take the maximum advantage of dietary fiber's protective effects, the ideal fiber consumption would be at least 45-50 grams per day. The sad reality is that in the United States the daily fiber intake is just a small fraction of the optimal values; it is estimated to be as little as 15 grams of fiber per day. The typical American diet doesn't contain much fiber. Highly processed foods are mainly composed of starch, sugar, protein and fat. During food processing, the majority of the plant's fiber content will be lost.

Until the past century, civilization diseases were absent among populations living a traditional lifestyle in the developing countries. For example, the famous missionary doctor *Albert Schweitzer* was astonished to encounter no cases of cancer upon his arrival in Gabon in 1913.

Denis P. Burkitt, a surgeon who spent 20 years in Africa noticed that certain diseases were non-existent or extremely rare among those people who live in a natural environment. Burkitt proposed that coronary heart disease, certain types of cancer, appendicitis, obesity and diabetes are associated with low fiber intake. *Peter Cleave* pointed

Food item	Insulin index	fiber content, %
White bread	73	1.8
Whole-wheat bread	50	9.2
White rice, cooked	55	0.5
Brown rice, cooked	29	1.5
Apples	43	2.3
Bananas	59	2.6
Avocado	4	5.6
Oranges	44	2.4
Grapes	60	0.9
Coleslaw	20	2.0
Carrots	44	2.8
Peanuts	15	8.4
Walnuts	5	6.7
Beans, kidney	34	24.9
Lentils	42	10.7
Pumpkin	77	0.5
Peas, green	37	4.5
Cauliflower	48	2.0

Table 27.1. Insulin index and fiber content of various foods

out that many civilization diseases are caused by the over-consumption of white flour and refined sugar. Both Burkitt and Cleave were right. If we add a sedentary lifestyle and smoking to low fiber intake and the overconsumption of refined carbohydrates, we have the recipe for a complete disaster.

Refined sugar and white flour have to be eliminated from our everyday diet. Long-term consumption of refined carbohydrates is detrimental to our health. Without the protective effects of dietary fiber, refined sugar and white flour cause a continuous, low-grade inflammation in our body. Long years, decades of exposure to a continuous inflammation in our body manifests in certain diseases. In some people, the inflammation causes cancer, while in others it leads to coronary heart disease, stroke, diabetes, arthritis or any other civilization disease.

Our daily fiber requirements can be easily met by reverting to unprocessed natural food. Eradicate white flour from your diet. It contains quickly digestible starch and only a minimum amount of fiber. Use traditionally milled coarse flour from rye or ancient wheat varieties such as *Einkorn* or *Emmer*. To read more see *Wheat, the Cereal Killer* chapter.

Nonsticky, long-grained brown rice is also a good source of dietary fiber. *The Story of Rice* chapter explains how to choose the right rice variety.

All legumes, especially beans, are an excellent source of dietary fiber. The highest fiber containing varieties include *dark red kidney, navy* and *cranberry beans*. Besides beans, lentils and chickpeas have a high fiber content as well. Legumes are rich in valuable plant proteins. These proteins, combined with whole grains, supply most of our essential amino acid requirements and are a good alternative for meat.

Kale is one of the world's healthiest foods, the cornerstone of a healthy diet. Besides fibers it contains antioxidants, calcium and vitamins. Most importantly, kale has a remarkable blood sugar lowering effect. Kale attenuates the blood glucose spikes after the consumption of a carbohydrate meal.[87] There are several recipes on how to prepare kale. However, to enjoy the maximum health benefits of kale, it always has to be consumed raw; eat the whole leaves, or cut them into larger pieces. Under no circumstances should you turn kale into a liquid by using a blender. Kale is not available in every store. The good news is that kale is very easy to grow at home. The plant doesn't require too much heat, sunshine or water. It can be grown even in cold climate countries such as Canada.

Chia seed is one of the recently re-discovered mysterious, ancient super foods. The plant was cultivated by the Aztecs even in pre-Columbian times. The seeds contain one third fiber, another third fats, and a considerable amount of protein, minerals and vitamins. Chia is the best available plant source of *omega-3 fatty acids*.

By incorporating kale and legumes in our diet and switching to whole grain rice and cereals, most of our daily fiber requirement will be met. Our fiber intake can be further increased by occasional consumption of walnuts, almonds, peanuts, avocado, flaxseed, sunflower seeds and rolled oats. All fruits and vegetables contain more or less fiber.

28

HOW MUCH FRUIT DO WE NEED?

THERE IS SOMETHING FISHY HERE

In newspaper articles, pamphlets and on websites that provide dietary advice to the lay public, we quite often come across the diet tip telling us to eat more fruits and vegetables in order to lose weight. This statement is just as stupid as it looks. Let's use some common sense! How is it possible to lose weight by eating more food? Maybe our brilliant diet experts meant we should replace some junk food with fruits and vegetables? For example, instead of drinking a 320-calorie supersized Coke at McDonalds we should have 4 apples. This would make perfect sense.

The *Dietary Guidelines for Americans* 2010 Edition says:
"… intake of at least $2^{1/2}$ cups of vegetables and fruits per day is associated with a reduced risk of cardiovascular disease, including heart attack and stroke."

Let's apply some critical thinking. My ultimate goal is to remain unbiased. What are the main benefits of fruit consumption? Fruits are excellent sources of dietary fiber, antioxidants, vitamins and minerals. They are indispensable nutrients; nobody would dispute it. Normally, this is where the story ends. Nobody talks about the adverse health effects. Since the onset of the *Green Revolution*, agriculture heavily relies on the use of pesticides and synthetic fertilizers. Systemic pesticides are chemicals that are actually absorbed by a plant, and even if you wash or peel the fruit you will still ingest the residues of the chemicals.

Apart from that, let's assume you eat organic fruits with no chemicals. Here is another problem: there are more than 2,000 types of fruits around the world. How can we simply assume that all fruits are equally good? Why do we love fruits? Because they are so sweet.

The sweeter the fruits are the more we love them. Remember, we are sugar addicts. Which apple would you pick from the supermarket's shelf: the giant, red ones with a high-gloss finish and a super-sweet taste or the tiny little greenish-yellow ones with moderate sweetness that are sold at half the price? I guess most people would choose the red ones. Customers demand super-sweet tasting fruits. Those ones with natural sweetness simply wouldn't sell, so they are not available in stores.

There is a big problem with sweet fruits: their sugar content outweighs the nutritional value of the antioxidants, minerals, vitamins and fiber. Fructose makes up more than half of their total sugar. Although fructose doesn't increase blood sugar levels, it is the most fattening of all sugars. Therefore, fruits with a high sugar content, especially those that are low in fiber, should be avoided. These types of fruits have the highest glycemic and insulin index. For example, pineapples and other tropical fruits with very intense sweet tastes are not good for you. In contrast, fruits from temperate climate countries that have a low sugar content are much healthier.

Regular consumption of apples have numerous health benefits. Free radicals play an important role in the development of most diseases. Antioxidants prevent cells from the harmful effects of these free radicals. Apples are rich in flavonoids, a type of antioxidants. Flavonoids have a protective effect by reducing the risk for cardiovascular disease, type-2 diabetes, and certain types of cancer. Apples are rich in soluble fibers. After ingestion of carbohydrate-rich meals, soluble fibers slow down the rate of absorption, preventing sudden spikes in blood glucose levels. Care needs to be taken when selecting the right variety. Avoid those apples that have a very intensely sweet taste. High sugar content offsets their health benefits. Don't peel apples. A significant portion of the valuable nutrients is in the skin.

Bananas are a little bit tricky. Nutritionally, green and fully ripe bananas are like two completely different fruits. In green bananas, sugar makes up only 7 percent of total dry matter, in overripe bananas 88 percent of total dry matter is sugar. Fully ripe bananas are a high glycemic index food and they should be avoided. On the other hand, green bananas contain mainly resistant starch that is indigestible.

HOW TO EAT FRUITS

As we saw from the previous examples, the general advice "eat more fruits" turned out to be wrong. It greatly depends on the circumstances whether a certain fruit is good for our health or not. There are a few practical tips below on how to maximize the health benefits of your fruit consumption.

Avoid excessively sweet fruits. Most of the tropical fruits fall in this category. Sometimes there are huge differences between fruit varieties. Let's take grapes for example. While the most popular grapes may contain up to 16% of sugar, the sugar content of less sweet varieties is only one third of that. Again, the sugars offset the health benefits of fibers, antioxidants, minerals and vitamins.

The sugar content of fruits also depends on their ripeness. During the ripening process starches will be gradually converted into sugars. We can increase their health benefits if fruits are consumed before they reach full ripeness.

Always eat fruits raw. Cooked fruits are digested at a faster rate that will result in higher blood glucose levels. Besides, cooking kills the vitamins. Never serve fruits with a sugary syrup or cookies. *Compote* (cooked fruits is a sweet syrup) is often served with main dishes or as dessert in many countries. This is not a healthy choice. Fruit jams are very popular, especially among children. Unfortunately, making jam is like an assassination against the goodness preserved in fruits. Jams contain excessive amounts of sugar, up to two thirds of their weight.

Dried fruits have been produced for thousands of years. Raisins, dates, prunes, figs, apricots, peaches, apples and pears are the most popular ones. Some fruits such as strawberries and mango are infused with sugar syrup prior to drying. Candied fruit is made by boiling fruit pieces in a sugar syrup. Because of their concentrated sugar content, dried and candied fruits are not recommended. We should eat fresh fruit instead.

Fruit juices definitely fall in the junk food category. They contain mostly sugar, acid, artificial flavor, coloring and additives. Manufacturers sometimes add some negligible amounts of "real" fruit just to cover up the junk components. What about 100% fruit juices? The problem is that during processing, a considerable amount of fiber is lost. Without the protective effect of fiber, the sugar content of the fruit will cause a sudden spike in blood glucose and insulin levels. Besides, real fruits don't have as intense flavor as expected. Manufacturers need to tune up the taste of their product with artificial flavors.

We can conclude that we should avoid fruits that have a very intensely sweet taste. Those varieties with a moderate sugar content are recommended up to two or three servings a week. Only apples should be a part of our everyday diet. Regular apple consumption improves glycemic control and prevents many diseases. The lowest possible sugar content is the most important point when choosing varieties. The high *soluble fiber* content of fruits further increases their health benefits.

Readers may ask the question: if we don't eat at least $2^{1/2}$ cups of fruits per day, as the *Dietary Guidelines* say, how do we meet our fiber, vitamin, mineral and antioxidant requirements? The answer is simple: from whole grains and vegetables. The good news is that they don't contain a lot of sugar and you can eat as much vegetables as you want.

29

VEGETABLES

EAT AS MUCH AS YOU WANT

Fruits and vegetables are an excellent source of a whole range of essential nutrients. The *Dietary Guidelines for Americans* 2010 Edition recommends the consumption of at least $2^{1/2}$ cups of vegetables and fruits per day. The problem with this approach is that it doesn't take into consideration sugar's adverse health effects: the relatively high sugar content of fruits outweighs the benefits of their valuable nutrients. On the other hand, vegetables are low in sugar, with a few exceptions. Vegetables contain all the necessary nutrients that fruits have, without a high sugar content. Therefore vegetables, and not fruits, should be our primary source of fiber, vitamins, minerals and antioxidants.

Legumes are an excellent source of dietary fiber. They are rich in valuable plant proteins. These proteins, combined with whole grains, supply most of our essential amino acid requirements and are a good alternative for meat. Peas and beans can be used for cooking as mature dried seeds or as green seeds together with the pods. During the ripening process the composition of these plants goes through significant changes: the protein and fiber content multiplies and sugar content decreases. Therefore, legumes in their mature form are more valuable than when eaten as green. Beans with a high fiber content, such as *dark red kidney*, *navy* and *cranberry beans* are the healthiest choices. Besides beans, other legumes such as peas, lentils and chickpeas are rich in fiber and proteins. Although, chickpeas are rich in nutrients, they also contain the highest amount of sugar of all legumes. Therefore the glycemic load of chickpeas is higher than of beans and lentils.

VEGETABLES

Leaf vegetables come from a very wide variety of plants. They are an indispensable part of a healthy diet. Leaf vegetables are high in dietary fiber and protein per calorie; they are also a good source of vitamins and minerals. Although there are many ways to prepare them, there are two basic principles we need to keep in mind. First, always eat leaf vegetables raw. Cooking increases their digestibility and impairs the protective effect of dietary fibers. Besides, a considerable amount of vitamins is lost during the cooking process. Second, eat the leaves whole, or cut into larger pieces. Don't turn them into a liquid by using a blender.

Kale is one of the world's healthiest foods, the cornerstone of a healthy diet. Besides fibers it contains antioxidants, calcium and vitamins. Most importantly, kale has a remarkable blood sugar lowering effect. Kale attenuates the blood glucose spikes after the consumption of a carbohydrate meal.[87] Kale has to be incorporated into our everyday diet and should be eaten as often and as much as possible.

Cabbage is high in dietary fiber and protein per calorie and is a rich source of vitamin C. It can be consumed either raw or cooked, however raw cabbage has more health benefits. Cabbage is a very efficient tool in a weight-loss diet, because it gives you the feeling of fullness quickly. Although cabbage, broccoli, cauliflower, kale, Brussels sprouts and kohlrabi look differently, they are just different cultivars of the same species. You can eat these vegetables as much as you want.

You can also eat those vegetables without limitations which have a *taproot*: carrot, parsley, radish, turnip and celery. However, beets have higher sugar content and they shouldn't be consumed in large quantities. The same rule applies to all kinds of vegetables: if they are edible in their raw form, they should be eaten raw.

Bulb vegetables, such as garlic, onion, leek and chives are rich in vitamins, minerals and antioxidants. Garlic is a universal remedy used for millennia. Garlic's health benefits include its blood pressure lowering, cardioprotective, antithrombotic, antimicrobial, antiinflammatory, and antioxidant effects. In addition, eating garlic can reduce the risk of developing several types of cancer.

Of the *nightshade* vegetables, tomatoes, peppers and eggplant are recommended. Those pepper varieties that have a higher sugar content (they are usually red and taste much sweeter than the others) shouldn't be eaten in large quantities. Some tomato varieties, especially those that are harvested fully ripe from the plant, have a high sugar content. In some cases it may be well over 6%, in contrast to an average 2% sugar content of regular tomatoes. Those very sweet tomatoes should be limited to one or two small pieces per serving. Avoid tomato in its processed forms such as paste, purée or ketchup because of the concentrated sugar content.

Cucumber can be eaten either fresh or pickled. Read labels carefully, sometimes pickles contain sugar. Those products should be blacklisted.

Squash varieties differ significantly in their nutrient composition. Those ones with high sugar content are not advised. *Bitter gourd* (Momordica charantia) is a member of the *gourd family*, a distant relative of squash, pumpkin and gourds. In India and China, it has been cultivated for centuries. Some authors reported that bitter gourd had a significant blood glucose lowering effect in both healthy subjects and diabetics.[88]

Mushrooms are delicious and contain valuable nutrients. They are a good source of protein, fiber, vitamins, minerals and antioxidants. Mushrooms can be eaten either cooked or raw. Mushrooms retain more of their valuable nutrients if they are not overcooked.

VEGETABLES THAT HAVE NO HEALTH BENEFIT

Sprouting has become very popular during the last decades. Germs of various plants such as soybean, barley, wheat, alfalfa, broccoli and many others are being sold by health stores claiming that sprout is a universal remedy capable of preventing and treating a whole range of diseases. It is often said that consumption of sprouts "boosts your immune system" and "increases enzymatic activity" and so on. Although sprouts contain high amounts of proteins, vitamins, minerals and other phytochemicals, the rest of those statements are not scientifically proven and such claims are often is mixed with pseudoscience. For example, *Ann Wigmore*, the main proponent of wheatgrass therapy was charged with healthcare fraud and quackery.

Despite the valuable nutrients, sprouts contain a certain enzyme, *amylase*, that breaks down starches into simple sugars. *Amylase* is the main enzyme component of malt, which is used by beer manufacturers. The pancreas and salivary glands in our body produce a sufficient amount of the amylase that is necessary for digestion. By adding high amylase content foods, such as sprouts, to our diet, we further increase the glycemic response to carbohydrate meals. A clinical study was done in Korea[89] to examine the alleged health benefits of barley sprouts. Subjects consumed one capsule of barley sprout extract a day for a period of 12 weeks. At the end of the experiment, barley sprout consumption showed no health benefits at all. Apart from a minimal improvement in their LDL cholesterol level, the lipid profile of the subjects got even worse. The fasting plasma glucose increased slightly and the plasma insulin increased significantly. In other words, barley sprout consumption not only showed zero health benefits, but it even turned out to be harmful.

Potatoes are the most consumed vegetable in the United States and in many countries around the world. Each American eats more than 119 pounds of potatoes every year. McDonald's alone buys 8% of the total amount of potatoes produced in the U.S. Potatoes are the perfect comfort food for many. Mashed potatoes, baked potatoes, boiled potatoes, roasted potatoes, French fries, potato chips and potato salad are very popular.

Potato consumption's proponents claim that potatoes are one of world's healthiest foods. It has no fat and contains vitamin C and B6 and potassium. Let's take a closer look at this claim that potatoes are really that good for us. What they won't tell you at McDonald's is that your French fries are made from potatoes that were treated with lots of harmful chemicals. Some of those pesticides are even carcinogenic (cancer-causing). According to the U.S. Department of Agriculture, 35 pesticide residues were found in potato samples.[90] Potato lovers don't know that before harvesting, the plants get sprayed with herbicides to kill off the green vines. Apart from pesticides, let's assume you eat organic potatoes. Are they really a healthy choice? I have bad news. Even if the cancer-causing chemicals are eliminated, there is still a big problem: potatoes are fattening.

Potatoes are starchy vegetables. Most of potato's dry matter is actually made up by starch. The French polymath, *Jean Anthelme Brillat-Savarin* established the fattening effect of starch 200 years ago. Unlike whole grains, potatoes are a very poor source of other nutrients. Compared to potatoes, whole grains contain 50% more protein and twice as much fiber, *as a percentage of dry matter*. Fiber is the main protective factor against sudden blood glucose and insulin spikes following a carbohydrate meal. Both potatoes and whole wheat contain a considerable amount of starch. However, the composition of these two types is totally different. Potato has a higher portion of rapidly digestible starch[91], which triggers a more severe insulin response than wheat starch. *Resistant starch* escapes digestion and it has numerous health benefits. Some experts argue that potatoes contain a high amount of resistant starch. Correct. Some potato varieties are exceptionally high in resistant starch. However, this is just a half truth. Cereals contain *type-1 resistant starch* that slows down digestion, especially if the kernels are ground into a coarse flour. Potatoes on the other hand have *type-2 resistant starch* that is even tougher than *type-1*, as potato lobbyists say. But after cooking potatoes, the starch is converted into its worst possible form that is absorbed rapidly, provoking quick glycemic response.[92] Blood glucose peaks are shortly followed by insulin spikes. For example, boiled potatoes have a twice as high insulin index as brown rice has.[93]

We can thus conclude, that potatoes have no valuable nutrients that can not be supplied from other sources. Because of their rapidly digestible starch component, frequent consumption of potatoes is not recommended. If you still can't live without them, limit your consumption to one serving per week. Boiled and mashed potatoes should be avoided. The best cooking method is frying in natural, cold pressed vegetable oil. Sweet potatoes, as their name suggests, are high in sugar and should be excluded from our diet.

30

DIETARY FAT

SATURATED FATS

Coronary heart disease was considered a very rare condition in the early 20th century. Parallel with the fast-paced economic growth in the 1960s however, cardiovascular disease had become a widespread epidemic that required quick action by the world's governments. Billions of dollars were spent on finding the cause of the number one threat to our health. New theories were born and old ones were neglected. The 150-year-old wisdom of the fattening effect of carbohydrates was quickly forgotten. Carbohydrates suddenly became a healthy food and dietary fat was declared to be the number one enemy of mankind. Saturated fats, the "wickedest" of all lipids, earned their especially bad reputation in the 1960s. The infamous pamphlet from 1977, entitled *Dietary Goals for the United States,* encouraged us to consume more carbohydrates and less fat. Unfortunately, people took the bad advice and did exactly what they were told to do: reduced their fat intake and increased their carbohydrate consumption. It is no wonder then, that the new dietary guidelines coincided with the beginning of the largest obesity epidemic in human history. Public policies toward fat consumption basically haven't changed since the 1970s. The *diet-heart hypothesis* is considered by mainstream scientists as a proven fact, rather than just a theory. The hypothesis says that dietary fat raises blood cholesterol and therefore increases the risk of coronary heart disease. In 1990, the *American Heart Association* (AHA) issued a scientific statement.[94] They identified saturated fatty acids, dietary cholesterol, and obesity as the main risk factors for heart disease. The authors argued that there is a "large body of evidence" proving the truth of the *diet-heart hypothesis.* Some researchers, including myself, took the time and did some in-depth investigation to verify whether that "large body of evidence" really exists. The studies cited in the AHA statement are very controversial. Some of the references are completely irrelevant, or the presented facts are exaggerated. The authors give too much weight to *Ancel Keys'* work. Mainstream scientists never mention the fact that one of the biggest skeptics of Keys' theory was Keys himself. Another important point is that some of the claims can not be even proven in humans, only by animal experiments. In addition to that, in one of the cited clinical trials researchers were even charged with fraud.[95]

Although the *diet-heart hypothesis* lacked that so-called "large body of evidence", it has still remained the only accepted theory by the vast majority of mainstream scientists even until today. Taking advantage of the weakness of the *diet-heart hypothesis*, alternative views started emerging in the beginning of the 1970s. *Robert Atkins*, was one of the most prominent early cholesterol deniers. From time to time, skeptics come up with even more absurd ideas then the original theory itself. For example, in 2012, the *British Journal of Nutrition* published a paper arguing that saturated fat consumption decreases the risk of dying from coronary heart disease.[96] Food intake and health statistics data were analyzed from 41 European countries including former Soviet republics. The author found that in Eastern Europe and in the former Soviet republics, where saturated fat intake is low, the prevalence of coronary heart disease is much higher than in Western Europe. A reconstructed graph is shown on Figure 30.1. For those who are familiar with the economics and geopolitics of the continent, it is obvious that France can not be compared to Azerbaijan. Former *Eastern Bloc* countries are substantially different from Western Europe concerning their economic situation, health care system, lifestyle and the dietary habits of their population. In addition to that, in the former Eastern Bloc countries food statistics are unreliable. Typically, food is not distributed in large supermarkets. A great number of the products are sold at farmers' markets, small stores, or are grown by people themselves. Such food data are not included in official statistics. If we take a second look at the graph, the bottom right area of the chart represents the Western European countries and the top left portion shows the former Eastern Bloc countries. Let's

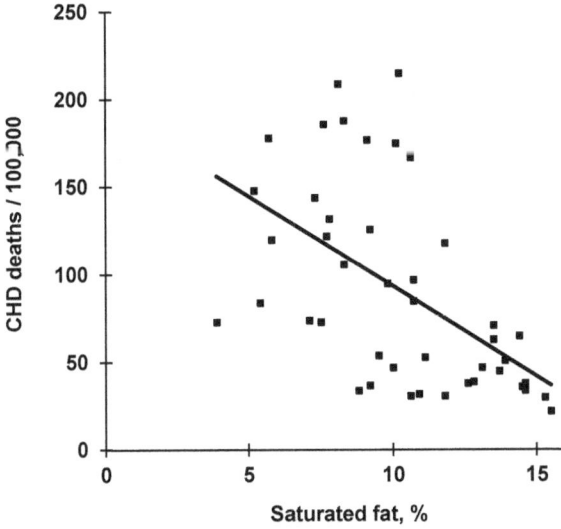

Figure 30.1. Misleading graph showing a strong negative correlation between saturated fat consumption and coronary heart disease death

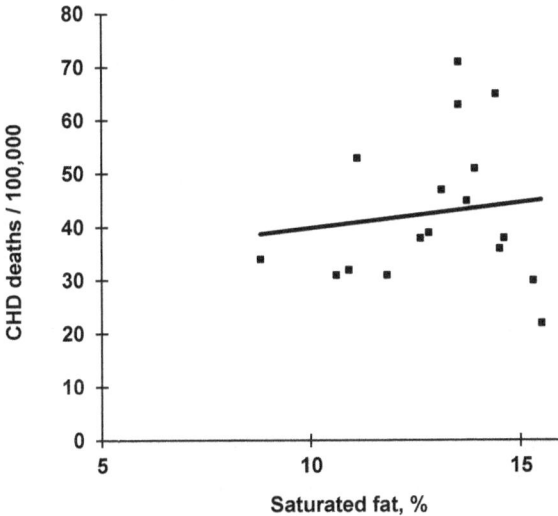

Figure 30.2. Western European countries show a weak positive correlation between saturated fat consumption and coronary heart disease death

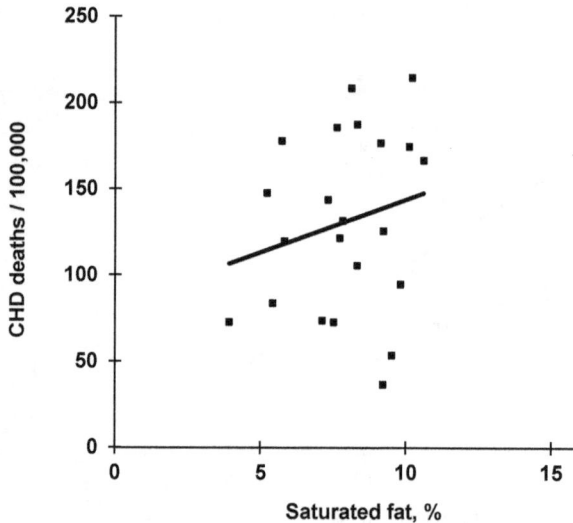

Figure 30.3. Eastern European countries show a weak positive correlation between saturated fat consumption and coronary heart disease death

draw a separate graph for the East, and another one for the West. Now, the trendline goes the opposite direction. Saturated fat just *slightly* increases the risk of coronary heart disease. See figures 30.2 and 30.3.

My main goal is to remain unbiased. I do not support either the skeptics or the mainstream scientists. Many studies show that there is still a very weak correlation between saturated fat consumption and heart disease. It is fairly less significant than mainstream researchers suggest, but cannot be completely ignored either, as the skeptics do.

It should be noted however, that very often the results even of the large clinical trials aren't very reliable. For example, a study was completed analyzing 1,042 cardiac events among 13,614 partici-pants.[97] In the experimental group, saturated fats were replaced with polyunsaturated fats (PUFA). Researchers found that based on the percentage of total energy consumption, every 5% replacement of saturated fats with PUFA reduced the coronary heart disease risk by 10%. The study was funded by the *National Heart, Lung, and Blood*

Institute, however a serious conflict of interest greatly undermines the study's credibility. If we read the fine print, one of the researchers was associated with pharmaceutical companies such as GlaxoSmithKline and Sigma Tau. It is very common that clinical trials are funded by the food or pharmaceutical industries. These days, such competing interests have to be disclosed by the authors of scientific papers, however that hasn't always been the case. Back in the 1960s and 70s when the foundations of the *diet-heart hypothesis* were laid, there were no such requirements and the industry-sponsored trials could not be identified.

A study that was sponsored by the *World Health Organization,* found that replacing each percent of saturated fat with 0.5% mono-unsaturated and 0.5% polyunsaturated fats resulted in approximately 0.06 mmol/l lower blood cholesterol levels.[98] Authors also **estimated** that one percent saturated fat reduction **would result** in 9,800 fewer coronary heart disease deaths and 3,000 fewer stroke deaths each year across all of the examined 15 European countries. I'd like to point out that the authors did not say that heart disease and stroke deaths *actually* decreased by such and such numbers as a result of saturated fat reduction. Rather, they are just **estimating the decrease** in the future **if** saturated fat consumption **would be** cut back by 1%. Such statements may be extremely misleading, especially if mainstream media takes them out of the original context.

There is a very common misconception that all saturated fats are harmful. This myth originated at the times of the vicious anti-fat campaign of the mass media. Most of the mainstream scientists agree that there are only three saturated fatty acids that can be associated with an increased risk of cardiovascular disease: *lauric, myristic* and *palmitic acid.* The rest of the saturated fatty acids are considered to be harmless.

In another study, subjects were put on a saturated fat diet containing high amounts of *lauric, myristic* and *palmitic acid.*[99] After three weeks, the LDL cholesterol level of the participants was found to be 0.47 mmol/liter higher compared to the other group who consumed monounsaturated fat. This 15% increase in LDL cholesterol levels looks pretty impressive, however if we read the fine print, we will see that the study was funded by *Sandoz Research Institute*, which belongs to *Novartis*, one of the largest pharmaceutical companies in the world.

The role of saturated fats in the development of cardiovascular disease remains a very controversial topic. A large number of clinical trials is sponsored by the pharmaceutical industry and only the positive findings are published. Medical journals regularly receive donations from pharmaceutical companies[66] that put a tremendous amount of pressure on the editors who decide which studies will be published and which ones will not. The results of unpublished trials and those that were published in smaller, independent journals supply a considerable amount of evidence that saturated fats play a significantly less important role in the development of cardiovascular disease than previously thought. Nevertheless, there is still a weak correlation between saturated fat intake and cardiovascular disease.

TRANS FATS

Trans fats, saturated fats and hydrogenated oils are often confused. Trans fats are one type of unsaturated fats, which have the hydrogen atoms on the opposite sides around the double bounds. Saturated fats have no double bonds. Both saturated and trans fats can cause adverse health effects. Now comes the real horror story. Naturally occurring, healthy unsaturated fats often fall prey to the junk food industry. The process is called *hydrogenation*, a chemical treatment of natural oils. Hydrogenation produces both saturated and trans fats. Hydrogenated oils are solid at room temperature and have an extended shelf life. Margarine, a completely artificial food, is manufactured from hydrogenated vegetable oils. Trans-fat-rich oils are also used in shortenings for deep-frying in restaurants. Hydrogenated trans fats increase the risk of coronary heart disease. Exceptionally, both mainstream scientists and cholesterol-skeptics agree.

In the previously mentioned experiment, besides saturated fats, trans fats were tested as well.[99]Researchers found that the LDL cholesterol level of those subjects who were on a diet rich in trans fats was 0.37 mmol/liter higher compared to the control group who consumed monounsaturated fats.

Although their harmful effects have been known for decades, industrially produced trans fats are still widely used. Ironically, nature also produces trans fats. The fat in beef, mutton and milk contains 2-8% trans fatty acids, which is formed by bacteria living in the stomach of ruminants (cows, sheep, goats, etc.). While some experts question the adverse health effect of naturally occurring trans fats, others consider natural and artificial trans fats equally harmful. It should be noted however, that trans fats in meat and milk occur in relatively small quantities and it is unlikely that these trans fats per se can be identified as a risk factor for cardiovascular disease. On the contrary, overconsumption of red meat and milk turned out to be harmful. How is it possible? We don't know the exact answer. These adverse health effects can be attributed to trans fats, saturated fats, total fat, proteins or other unknown factors as well.

UNSATURATED FATS

Monounsaturated fats have a proven LDL-cholesterol lowering effect. Olive oil is the best source of monounsaturated fatty acids, with an average 75% *oleic acid* content. Polyunsaturated fats have a similar protective effect against high LDL-cholesterol. Seed oils such as sunflower, safflower and sesame oil are very rich in *linoleic acid*. There are two essential fatty acids that cannot be produced by our body: *linoleic acid* and *linolenic acid.* Therefore, our diet must include sufficient amounts of these important fatty acids. Marine fish oils contain *long chain* and *very long chain* polyunsaturated fatty acids.

The terms *omega-3* and *omega-6* fatty acids are often used in the scientific literature. *Omega-3* means that the first double bound is located at the third place from the end of the molecule. In *omega-6* fatty acids the first double bound is at the sixth place. Special attention needs to be paid to the ratio of *omega-3* and *omega-6* fatty acids. Although *omega-6* fatty acids are very important, they can also be harmful when *omega-6* fatty acids are out of balance with *omega-3* fatty acids. Excess amounts of *omega-6* fatty acids are converted into *eicosanoids* that promote inflammation in our body. When *omega-3* fatty acids are abundant, fewer *omega-6* fatty acids are converted into proinflammatory *eicosanoids*. A whole range of civilization diseases is associated with continuous, low-grade inflammation in our body. Due to their anti-inflammatory properties, *omega-3* fatty acids serve as a powerful tool in the prevention of many modern-day diseases such as cardiovascular disease, stroke, arthritis, asthma, certain cancers, Alzheimer's disease and depression. It is estimated that in industrialized countries, the proportion of the consumed *omega-6* and *omega-3* fatty acids is between 10:1 and 15:1. The ideal ratio promoting health and longevity would be 4:1.[100] A westernized diet does not provide a sufficient amount of *omega-3* fatty acids. Japan is the only exception among the industrialized countries which has an adequate amount of *omega-3* fatty acid intake, due to the high fish consumption of the Japanese. The high amount of *omega-3* fatty acids in the traditional Japanese diet is correlated with the exceptionally low prevalence rate of obesity and cardiovascular disease in Japan, compared to other developed countries.

Modern agriculture and farming techniques don't favor healthy fatty acid composition. To achieve quick growth, animals are fed with concentrates beside being treated with hormones. A study was done in Brazil to compare the quality of traditional, grass-fed beef with grain-fed beef.[101] Researchers found that the ratio of *omega-6* and *omega-3* fatty acids was significantly better in grass-fed beef compared to grain-fed beef (3.6:1 and 5.8:1, respectively). An Australian study showed a 2 to 3 fold increase in 18:1 *trans fats*, comparing beef from grain-fed and grass-fed animals.[102]

ANIMAL FATS

Dietary guidelines suggest that we should eat less animal fat. Mainstream scientists associate animal fat consumption with high blood cholesterol levels and an increased risk for coronary heart disease. They argue that saturated fatty acids abundantly found in animal products are one of the main contributory factors to cardiovascular disease. Some media health experts even use the terms *animal fat* and *saturated fat* interchangeably. Let's take a quick look at the fatty acid composition of animal fats. There are differences among species, but generally, about half of the fat content of domestic animals is made up of saturated fatty acids. The other half is composed of mostly monounsaturated fatty acids and a small amount of polyunsaturated fatty acids. There are only three saturated fatty acids that can be considered potentially harmful: *lauric*, *myristic* and *palmitic acid*. These three together are the "bad" ones that make up about one quarter of the total fat content. In other words, three quarters of the fatty acids in animal fat is good, or at least neutral.

Some cholesterol skeptics take advantage of the lack of strong scientific evidence against saturated fats and they claim that animal fats are a healthy, natural choice. They often encourage people to refrain from lean meat and use animal fat for cooking instead of vegetable oils. There are two big problems however. First, there is no scientific evidence at all, supporting the claim that animal fats are any healthier than vegetable oils. Second, mainstream scientists lack the proof of their theory as well. There is just a very weak correlation between saturated fat intake and cardiovascular disease.

In my opinion, we shouldn't worry too much about the fat that *naturally* occurs in meat products. Foods made from lean meat usually contain sugar, which is much worse than any kind of fat. On the other hand, don't use animal fat for cooking. Animal fats have zero health benefits. Prepare your meals with cold pressed vegetable oils instead.

VEGETABLE OILS

Care should be taken when choosing the right oil for cooking. Traditionally made organic oils are nutritious and are an excellent source of essential fatty acids, antioxidants and certain vitamins. When shopping for the right oil, there are a few things to consider. Completely avoid any food items made from genetically modified organisms. The global market share of GMO crops is increasing each year. Actually the globalization went so far that in certain countries it is already hard to find non-GMO versions of certain plants. In the United States for example, the vast majority of the corn and soy crops are genetically modified. The long-term health effects of genetically modified foods are unknown. Although genetically modified foods are declared to be safe by health authorities, don't take it at face value. We should keep in mind that scientific research is directly or indirectly funded by the food and pharmaceutical industry. As a general rule, only trials with positive outcomes are published. Those studies interfering with Big Pharma and Big Food are silenced very quickly. For example, Hungarian biochemist and nutritionist *Árpád Pusztai*, who spent 36 years at the *Rowett Research Institute* in Aberdeen, Scotland was fired for pointing out that genetically modified potatoes are harmful. Pusztai's research data were seized and he was banned from speaking publicly.

Apart from GMO foods, here is another horror story. Besides regular pesticides, *Glyphosate* is sprayed on certain crops to speed up harvest (for example on sunflower). The *International Agency for Research on Cancer*, classified Glyphosate as a probable carcinogen (cancer causing) chemical.

At the processing plant, the oil content is extracted from the seeds by applying heat, pressure and chemical solvents. Then, the "crude oil" goes into the refinery. In this step, proteins, vitamins, pigments and other "impurities" are removed by further mechanical and chemical processes. As a final step, the oil gets bleached and deodorized.

In conclusion, we should avoid every kind of refined, unnatural vegetable oil. Only those products are recommended that are produced by cold pressing from organically grown plants.

Canola oil is probably the most controversial of all vegetable oils. The product earned the *Heart-Check Certificate* of the *American Heart Association*. Besides the AHA certificate, there are a few other good reasons as well to completely avoid canola oil. Proponents of canola argue that the oil contains low levels of saturated fatty acids and has an optimal ratio of *omega-3* and *omega-6* fatty acids. This part is correct. However, the rest of the story is not printed on the labels. Canola oil is a typical example of engineered food. The oil is extracted from oilseed rape, which was originally an inedible plant because of its high content of toxic *erucic acid*. Decades of selective breeding techniques resulted in *double zero* cultivars, which contain a significantly lower amount of toxic substances. This is not all. In 1995 *Monsanto* introduced the new, genetically modified canola. The new, GMO canola is *Roundup ready*. What this term basically means is that the crops can be sprayed with even more herbicide without killing the plant itself.

THE GOOD OILS

As discussed earlier, maintaining the correct ratio of *omega 6* and *omega-3* fatty acids is very important. Our goal is to intake as much *omega-3* fatty acids as we can, and to minimize the consumption of *omega-6* fatty acids. The ideal ratio is no more than 4 parts of *omega-6* fatty acids for each part of *omega-3* fatty acids. Fatty sea fish are a rich source of long chain and very long chain *omega-3* fatty acids. Flaxseed oil is the best plant source for *omega-3* fatty acids. Natural flaxseed oil starts to break down when exposed to air or high temperatures. Therefore, it has to be stored refrigerated, and can not be used for frying or cooking. Flaxseed oil should be the number one choice for salad dressings, cold dishes and any other applications that don't require heating the oil. Chia is a newly rediscovered super food. More than half of its oil content is *omega-3*; it is also an excellent source of dietary fiber and protein. Chia oil for food is not available in stores. Chia seeds are eaten raw. Soak them in water half an hour before your meal.

Fish oil, flaxseed oil and chia seeds are the main concentrated sources of *omega-3* fatty acids that are also low in *omega-6* fatty acids. There are some other sources of *omega-3* fatty acids as well, but their *omega-6:omega-3* ratio is significantly higher. I'd like to emphasize that for those foods that don't require heating the oil, *flaxseed oil* should be the number one choice. For anything else, use cold pressed extra virgin olive oil. The total *omega-6* fatty acid content of olive oil is not too high. The *omega-3* ratio can be easily fixed with additional intake of fish oils, flaxseed oil and chia seeds. By adding these food items to your everyday diet, you will enjoy the maximum health benefits of a balanced, healthy diet rich in *omega-3* fatty acids. Once in a while, you can also use other natural, cold pressed vegetable oils as well. Occasionally, you may also eat nuts and other oily seeds. Palm oil and coconut oil don't offer any health benefits because they have an exceptionally high saturated fatty acid content – even three times as much as animal fats do.

31

ANIMAL PROTEINS

INCREASING MEAT CONSUMPTION

In developing countries, meat consumption has been steadily increasing over the last half a century. Among the industrialized nations however, meat eating peaked in the early 2000s and since then, it has been continuously declining. In the economically less developed countries, meat is considered as a symbol of affluence. As a country's wealth grows, so does its meat consumption. Traditional eating patterns are gradually replaced with Western food that contains high amounts of refined carbohydrates and meat. China is one of the world's fastest growing markets. As a result of wealth accumulation in urban areas, China's middle class is exploding. As an alternative to traditional Chinese values, the Western lifestyle continues to gain more popularity, especially among the youth. McDonald's is still an undeniable symbol of the American lifestyle. In 2017, McDonald's announced plans to double the number of its restaurants in China within five years.

As traditional food is gradually replaced with Western food and meat consumption increases, so does the prevalence of Western diseases that were rare in economically less developed countries. For example, coronary heart disease, cancer and diabetes have been rising at an alarming rate in developing countries. Figure 31.1 shows the increasing per capita meat consumption since 1990 in China, South Korea, Brazil and Mexico. Although South Korea is a highly industrialized country, the occurrence of civilization diseases follows the same pattern as the other three countries. Parallel with meat consumption, the prevalence of ischemic heart disease, cancer and diabetes is steadily increasing (See Figures 31.2 , 31.3 and 31.4). Meat consumption is definitely correlated to Western diseases.

Meat Consumption

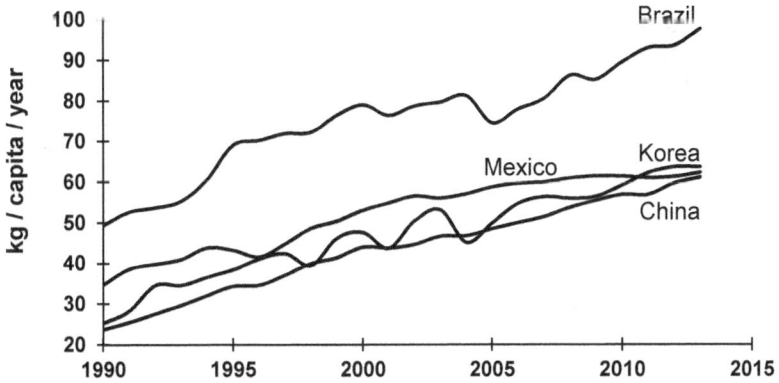

Figure 31.1. Per capita meat consumption in four countries

Ischemic Heart Disease

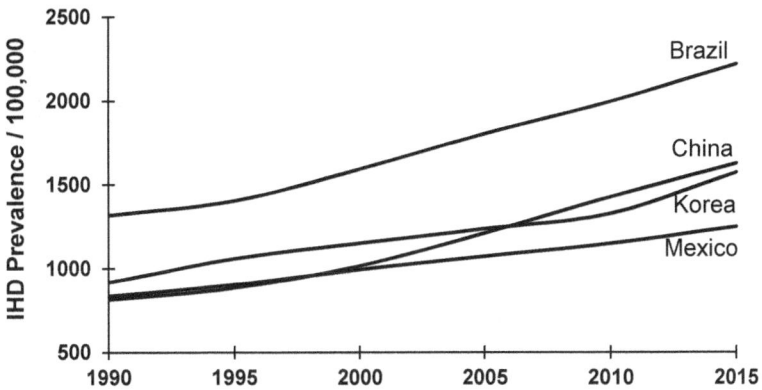

Figure 31.2. Prevalence rates of ischemic heart disease

Cancer Prevalence

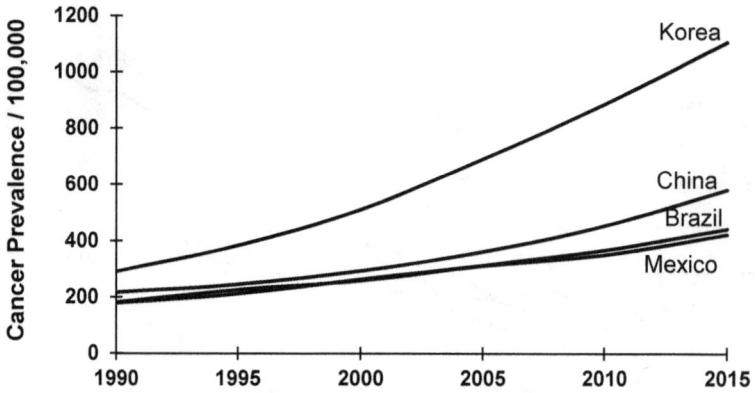

Figure 31.3. Cancer prevalence rates

Diabetes Prevalence

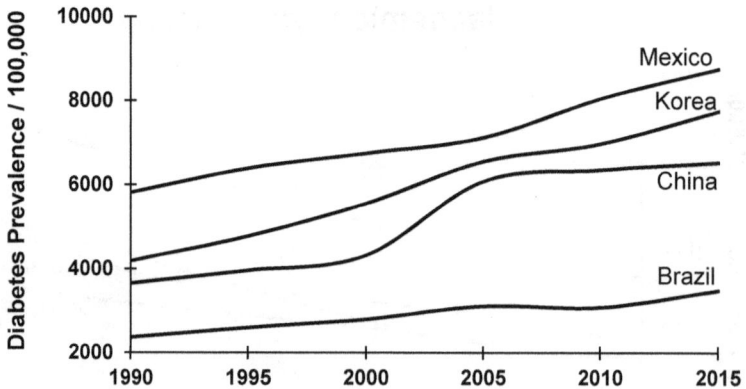

Figure 31.4. Diabetes prevalence rates

Correlation however, doesn't necessarily mean causation. I am not saying that high meat consumption is the only possible cause of our modern-day diseases, but rather that it is one of the major contributing factors. Although low fiber intake, highly refined carbohydrate consumption and physical inactivity also play an important role in the development of many diseases, the consequences of high meat consumption should not be neglected.

WHAT'S WRONG WITH MEAT?

I am not trying to convince anybody to become a vegetarian. However, the central role of meat in our diet needs to be re-evaluated. There are two problems with our dietary habits: the amount and the quality of meat that we consume. The average meat consumption in Western countries is estimated between 200 and 250 pounds per person annually. To have that much meat, we need to eat a third of a cow, or 62 chickens. In contrast, the Japanese, who are much healthier than Westerners, eat only 110 pounds of meat each year. *Blue Zones* are regions of the world where people live much longer than average. Such areas include Sardinia in Italy, Icaria in Greece and Okinawa in Japan. What is the common feature in the diet of Blue Zone people? They live on a predominantly plant-based diet and eat meat only occasionally. Westerners eat significantly more meat and they are also much sicker than people throughout the Blue Zones regions of the world.

The second problem is the quality of meat. What is wrong with commercially produced meat? The answer is: everything from the first step to the last step. Modern agriculture and farming techniques don't really produce healthy food at all. To achieve quick growth, animals are fed with concentrates instead of letting them graze naturally. In the previous chapter, we have discussed that grass-fed beef has a significantly better *omega-6:omega-3 fatty acid* ratio compared to grain-fed beef. Raising livestock the natural way greatly improves the quality of various animal products.

To promote faster growth, synthetic versions of naturally occurring sex hormones such as *testosterone* and *progesterone* are used in beef production. In addition to sex hormones, animals are also treated with *xenobiotic* substances that do not occur naturally in living organisms. Although the United States is the main market for hormone-raised beef, because of growing health concerns, the use of hormones in meat production is no longer allowed in the European Union.

As a result of the cholesterol hysteria starting in the 1970s, lean meat products became a symbol of healthier food choices. To make their products more appealing to customers, food manufacturers add a considerable amount of sugar to their "heart healthy" low-fat meat products. As previously discussed, sugar is much more harmful that fat. Consumption of excessive amounts of refined carbohydrates is the main driving force behind a whole range of modern-day civilization diseases.

The United States is one of the largest red meat consumers in the world. Results of the latest research associated red meat consumption with an increased risk of serious disorders such as *metabolic syndrome*[103], *cardiovascular disease*[104], *cancer*[104] and *diabetes.*[105] Red meat products contain larger quantities of *heme iron*, which under certain circumstances plays an important role in the formation of *free radicals* causing oxidative stress. This condition leads to a continuous low-grade inflammation in the body, which is associated with a whole range of diseases.

In Western countries a large amount of meat is consumed not in its natural state but in a highly processed form such as hot dogs, hamburgers, sausages, salami, canned meat, etc. Processed meat turned out to be even more harmful than red meat.[106] During processing, meat is exposed to various chemicals such as nitrates, nitrites, phosphates and smoke.

THE SOLUTION

It is almost impossible to stay healthy by eating such large amounts of artificially processed meats, the equivalent of one third of a cow or 62 chickens every year. Processed meat is the most harmful of all animal products, therefore it should be completely eliminated. White meat is a much healthier choice than red meat. Beef contains hormones, heme iron, trans fats and has a bad omega-6:omega-3 ratio. If you can't live without it, it should be eaten only in small amounts on special occasions; no more than once a week. However, the best option is not eating red meat at all. Poultry and fish are perfect substitutes for red meat.

As discussed previously, I argue that we need to reconsider the central role of meat in our diet. People in wealthy countries, as a symbol of affluence, tend to consume much more meat than their body really needs. The healthiest and longest-living people in the world eat meat only once or twice a week. This is one of their secrets of health and longevity. An average American eats 5 pounds of meat every weak. This is way too much *heme iron*, hormone residual, omega-6 fatty acid and food preservatives. Try to limit your weekly meat intake to a maximum of 1 to 1.5 pounds. This amount can be served in small daily portions or 2 - 3 larger meals a week. Prepare your meat the way you like. You don't need to worry too much about fat naturally occurring in meat. For cooking, use extra virgin, cold-pressed olive oil. Don't use flour or sugar for gravies and sauces.

Fish is healthier than meat. Try to replace meat with fish in your diet. Fatty sea fish are a rich source of omega-3 fatty acids. Eat any fish you like with two exceptions. Completely avoid fish preserved by salting. You can salt fish moderately, but commercially produced salted fish may contain up to 20% salt. The consumption of that much salt is unhealthy. This salt content is about 5-10 times higher than normal. As for canned fish, always read labels. Avoid junky ingredients like sugar, or GMO soy oil. Buy canned fish in spring water. Drain the water and add two tablespoons of flaxseed oil on the fish. This will make your perfect omega-3 day.

PLANT PROTEINS

Plant proteins are a healthy alternative to meat. All the necessary amino acids that are present in meat can be supplied from plant foods as well. There are 20 naturally-occurring amino acids, and 10 of them are called essential, which means the body can not synthesize them. There are only four so-called *limiting amino acids* that have a particular importance in the protein synthesis in our body: *lysine, methionine, threonine* and *tryptophan*. With regular consumption of whole grains and legumes, we can easily meet our essential amino acid requirements.

EGG CONSUMPTION

Thanks to the worldwide epidemic of cholesterol hysteria, egg consumption in the United States has been declining since the 1970s. You shouldn't worry too much about dietary cholesterol because it has just a negligible effect on LDL cholesterol levels. [73, 107] Cholesterol is present in almost every single cell of our body as a building block of the cell membrane. Cholesterol is also an important component of bile and is the raw material of vitamin D and various hormones. Literally, there is no life without cholesterol. Every single day, our body synthesizes approximately 700 milligrams of cholesterol. The more cholesterol you eat, the less cholesterol your body has to produce.

Although eggs are high in cholesterol, egg consumption doesn't significantly affect blood cholesterol levels. You can safely eat eggs without worrying about your blood cholesterol levels.

The quality of eggs greatly depends on the circumstances in which the animals are kept. Eggs laid by free-range chickens are more nutritious than the eggs of caged animals fed with commercial hen mash. Eggs from pastured chickens are rich in vitamin A and have twice as high vitamin E and omega-3 fatty acid content compared to caged chickens in commercial farms.

32

MILK AND DAIRY

WE WERE TOLD TO DRINK MORE MILK

The 2015 *Dietary Guidelines For Americans* recommends the consumption of 3 cups of milk a day for adults. *Canada's Food Guide* goes even further: teenagers are supposed to have 3 to 4 cups of milk every day. The alleged health benefits of milk include reducing the risk of osteoporosis, cardiovascular disease, cancer, osteoarthritis, diabetes, depression and the list goes on. Unfortunately, none of these claims can be proven. The evidence supporting milk's health benefits is scarce. There is conflicting research data, and the evidence proving the negative health effects of milk and dairy products is as plentiful as those showing health benefits.

IS MILK REALLY GOOD FOR YOU?

Osteoporosis is a disease that is associated with a decrease in bone density making the bones fragile. Since calcium is the main mineral in bone tissue and dairy products are high in calcium, it was also assumed that milk consumption actually protects against osteoporosis. Let's see if milk really protects us from osteoporosis? The role of dairy consumption in the prevention of osteoporosis has been studied for decades, however the results are very controversial. There are numerous studies showing that dairy products have a protective effect against osteoporosis. On the contrary, others found that dairy consumption doesn't prevent bone fractures at all, or milk is even detrimental to bone health.

A 12-year prospective study was done with the participation of 77,761 female registered nurses. The participants were put into four classes based on their milk consumption. The frequency of hip and forearm fractures was analyzed by statistical methods. Surprisingly, the lowest numbers of bone fractures occurred among those who consumed the lowest amount of dairy products. The study found that it is unlikely that a high consumption of milk protects against hip and forearm fractures.[108]

Based on hip fracture and dairy consumption statistics from 37 countries[109], there is a strong correlation (r=0.84) between milk consumption and the prevalence of hip fractures (see Figure 32.1). Although correlation doesn't necessarily mean causation, I'd like to point out the fact that countries with a high dairy consumption have the highest hip fracture rates as well. The role of milk consumption in the development of cancer is even more controversial. Some studies show a positive association, while others show a negative relationship between dairy intake and the development of various cancers. For example, a Norwegian prospective study with 15,914 participants found a strong relationship between milk consumption and the

Milk Consumption - Hip Fractures

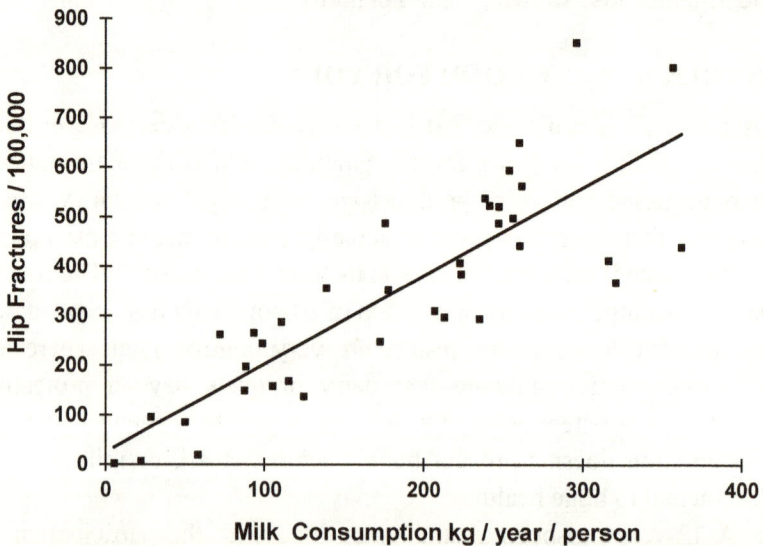

Figure 32.1. The correlation of milk consumption and hip fractures

184

cancers of the lymphatic organs (odds ratio: 3.4).[110] Many other cancers were found to be associated with milk consumption as well. On the other hand, milk showed a protective effect against bladder cancer.

Milk naturally contains a certain hormone, called *insulin-like growth factor-1* (IGF-1). Humans also produce IGF-1; the hormone stimulates cell growth, affecting almost every cell of our body. Besides its growth promoting effect, IGF-1 also contributes to the proliferation of cancer cells. Milk consumption may increase serum IGF-1 levels by up to 23%, especially in non-Caucasian individuals.[111] Dairy cows in the United States and a few other countries are treated with *bovine somatotropin* hormone, to increase milk productivity. Milk from hormone-treated animals may contain up to 83% more IGF-1.[112] High IGF-1 levels are associated with an increased risk for certain cancers.

Lactose is the major carbohydrate in milk. Fluid milk has a 4-5% lactose content on average. Lactose-intolerant people lack the enzyme *lactase* that digests the milk sugar. In the absence of lactase, after ingestion of milk, lactose passes undigested into the colon and is fermented by gut bacteria. Symptoms may include abdominal pain, bloating, diarrhea and nausea. Following the first few months of life, lactase activity starts to decrease. After weaning, in many individuals lactase activity declines to undetectable levels.

The prevalence of lactose intolerance greatly varies among different populations. In Northern European countries about 10% of the people are lactose intolerant. About half of Southern Europeans and the majority of Chinese suffer from lactose intolerance.

CASEIN IS THE MAIN CULPRIT

Casein makes up 80% of milk's protein content. Under certain circumstances, casein acts as a carcinogenic agent. Dr. T. Colin Campbell in his book *The China Study*, speaks about the tumor-promoting effect of casein. In experimental animals, the growth of tumor cells can be simply turned on or off by administering or withdrawing casein. A recent study found that casein promotes the proliferation of human prostate cancer cells as well.[113]

As we previously discussed, the role of milk in the development of civilization diseases is controversial. Some studies link milk to a whole range of disorders, while others show the health benefits of milk consumption. When evaluating the connection between milk and various health conditions, researchers traditionally focused on total milk consumption only, or on a main nutrient group of milk such as protein, lactose or fatty acids. Research data on the health impact of individual milk proteins was scant until the 1990s. Professor *Bob Elliott* from *Auckland University* discovered that there is a ten-fold difference in the incidence of type-1 diabetes among Samoan children living in New Zealand compared to Samoan children living in Samoa. Elliott noticed that in New Zealand the milk is rich in a specific protein, called *A1 beta-casein*. This particular protein leads to systemic inflammation and gastrointestinal disorders similar to those of lactose intolerance.

With the introduction of modern farming techniques, traditional breeds were replaced with *Holstein* cattle. Since *Holstein* cows are exceptionally productive they are the dominant dairy cow breed in industrialized countries. In the United States, 94 percent of dairy cows are of *Holstein* descent. Needless to say, the highly productive *Holstein* cows produce milk that contains the harmful *A1 beta-casein*. The milk of less popular European breeds like *Guernsey* or Asian and African breeds such as *Zebu* don't contain *A1 beta-casein*. The milk of other species, for example sheep, goat or camel is free of *A1 beta-casein*.

In the gastrointestinal tract, *A1 beta-casein* brakes down into *beta-casomorphin 7* (BCM7), which is a strong opioid. BCM7 is a risk factor for the development of life-threatening diseases, including type-1 diabetes and cardiovascular disease. In many individuals, the enzyme DPP4 prevents *casomorphin* from entering the bloodstream, while in others, *casomorphin* through the blood may get into the brain. BCM7 in the brain causes behavior patterns similar to those observed in autism and schizophrenia.

Based on milk consumption data from 48 countries, a strong correlation was found between the prevalence rates of type-1 diabetes and the amount of consumed milk per person (r=0.7). See Figure

32.2. Elliott found a very strong correlation (r=0.98) between *beta-casein* (A1 + B) consumption and diabetes.[114] I'd like to emphasize that r=0.98 means an exceptionally strong correlation between two variables. Even Ancel Keys' "doctored" diagram showed a weaker relationship, an r value of 0.96 between dietary fat intake and heart disease death rates. A study was done in Finland, with the participation of healthy siblings of children with type-1 diabetes.[115] Researchers analyzed the relationship between milk consumption of healthy children and the risk of becoming diabetic. Those children, who consumed over 540 ml of milk daily, were five times more likely to develop diabetes.

Milk Consumption and Diabetes

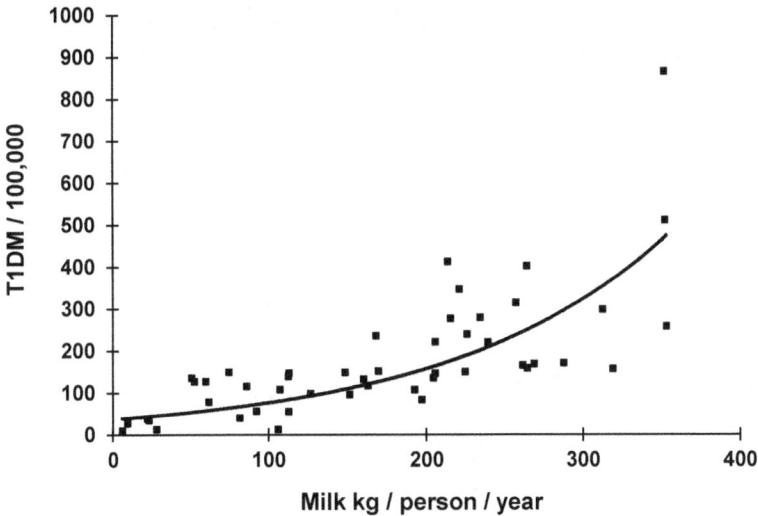

Figure 32.2. The correlation of milk consumption and type-1 diabetes

THE COW AND THE CORONARY

Milk's fatty acid composition is far from ideal: the trio of the "bad" saturated fatty acids (C12-C16) make up a third of the total fatty acid content. Milk also contains up to 4% trans fat. Hardcore fat-fanatics blame the detrimental health effects on milk's fat content. *Casein*, however turned out to be even more harmful than fat. Based on milk consumption data from 52 countries, there is just a moderate correlation (r=0.32) between milk consumption and ischemic heart disease deaths. *Beta-casein A1* intake and heart disease however, are highly correlated (r=0.63, see Figure 32.3). Although the negative health effect of *beta-casein A1* is supported by statistical data, the exact mechanism of how casein increases the risk of coronary heart disease is not entirely understood. It is assumed that *beta-casomorphin 7,* that is a byproduct of casein's digestion, plays an important role in the pathogenesis of heart disease. *Peptic ulcer* was traditionally treated with milk, by using the so-called "Sippy diet". In 1960, a paper was published about the alarmingly high rate of heart attack among those

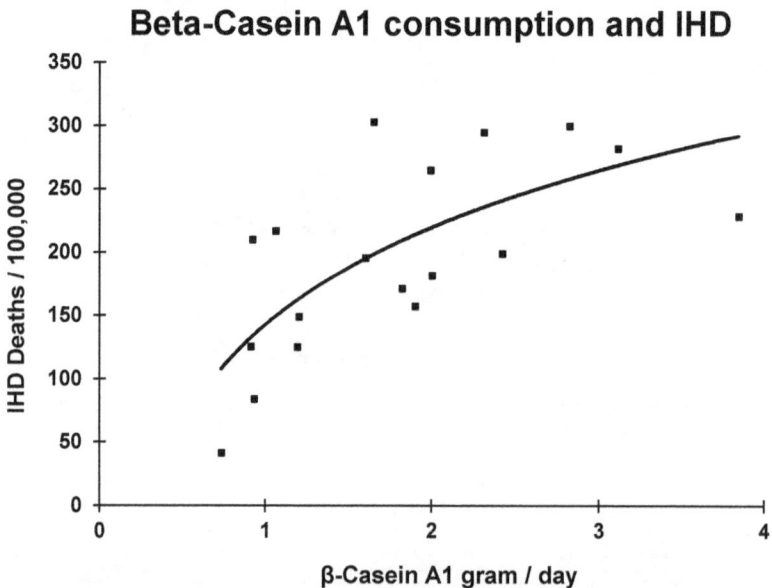

Figure 32.3. Beta-casein A1 consumption and the death rates of ischemic heart disease

who suffered from peptic ulcer and were treated with a milk diet. In Britain, those with peptic ulcers and who were consuming milk, were six times as likely to have a heart attack, compared to those who suffered from ulcers and didn't drink milk. In the United States, those ulcer patients that consumed milk were 2.4 times more likely to have a heart attack compared to those who didn't drink milk.[116] People with stomach ulcers have a damaged digestive system, therefore in their body *beta-casomorphin 7* is capable of freely entering the bloodstream. *Beta-casomorphin 7* is a strong opioid and also shows atherogenic properties (which causes the development of plaque in the arteries). It is assumed that BCM7 promotes the formation of plaques on the arterial walls; therefore is a risk factor for coronary heart disease.

THE CASE AGAINST COW MILK

Many of you might have heard notions like "Milk is for babies only" or "Humans are the only species on the earth that consume the milk of other species". The second statement needs a little correction: in some countries, cats and other domestic animals drink milk as well. As for the first sentence, I completely agree. Adults and big kids simply don't need milk. In its form, fake cow milk that is available on supermarket shelves is far more harmful than nutritious. What's wrong with milk? Everything from the first step to the last step.

During the last century, in many countries *Holstein* cattle gradually displaced traditional breeds. *Holstein is* exceptionally productive, however the cows' milk contains *beta-casein A1,* which may cause a series of health conditions in sensitive individuals.

In industrialized countries, traditional farming techniques were replaced with new concepts. Instead of grazing, cows are fed with concentrates. Unnatural feeding technology alters the fatty acid composition of the milk. On the contrary, traditionally produced, milk of grass-fed cows has a significantly better omega-6:omega-3 fatty acid ratio and is rich in *conjugated linoleic acid.*

Dairy cows in the United States and a few other countries are treated with *bovine somatotropin* hormone, to increase milk productivity. Due to several health concerns, milk from hormone-treated animals is banned in Canada and the European Union.

Pasteurization of milk has been mandatory in the industrialized countries for almost a century. It is a well-known fact that heat treatment impairs the availability of vitamins; particularly vitamin B2 and vitamin B12 levels in pasteurized milk are virtually zero. Manufacturers try to fix this problem by adding artificial vitamins to milk. Besides the vitamin loss, there is a bigger issue with it as well. Pasteurization of milk significantly increases the risk of cardiovascular disease. Over half a century ago, *J. C. Annand* did an in-depth analysis on how the introduction of mandatory milk pasteurization in the United Kingdom affected the occurrence of cardiovascular and cerebrovascular events. Annand compared the prevalence rates of the diseases before and after the introduction of pasteurization. He found that angina pectoris mortality increased by 82% in the United Kingdom, and in London by 261%. Cerebral embolism and thrombosis mortality increased by 42% in the UK.[117] It is assumed that prolonged heat treatment of milk protein may be an important factor in the pathogenesis of cardiovascular disorders.

Health authorities prohibit raw milk sales in many countries. They argue that raw milk is unsafe, therefore it needs to be pasteurized to kill harmful bacteria. This is true for milk coming from "cow factories" only, where the cows rarely graze and are fed with concentrates. The animals are kept in dirty, crowded spaces. In such unhealthy environments cows often get sick and are treated with hormones and antibiotics. On the contrary, the production of organic, grass-fed raw milk in the United States is strictly regulated. Animals are kept very clean and all cows must be examined by a veterinarian. The milk from different animals is collected separately. This kind of milk doesn't contain harmful bacteria.

In Western countries most of the commercially sold milk is homogenized. Homogenization is a physical process of pushing milk under high pressure through a tiny orifice. Homogenization reduces the size of the fat globules in milk. The process prevents cream from separating and rising to the top of the bottle. Homogenization increases the number and surface area of the fat globules. As a result of larger surface area, molecules are exposed to oxygen, and nutrients become more easily oxidized. Compared to pasteurization, homogenization causes significantly less damage or no damage to milk's ingredients. Nevertheless, unhomogenized milk is recommended over homogenized milk.

As a result of the cholesterol and fat hysteria started in the 1970s, milk is typically sold as reduced-fat or low-fat milk. Like always, we were given bad advice. Skim milk is actually more harmful than whole milk. Fats slow down the digestion of carbohydrates; therefore whole milk has a significantly lower insulin index than skim milk. As discussed earlier, some milk proteins, such as *A1 beta-casein* are detrimental to our health. Milk with a higher fat content is relatively lower in casein compared to skim milk and is considered to be less harmful.

PRACTICAL ADVICE

Milk was meant for babies. Adults simply don't need milk. It doesn't contain any specific nutrient that cannot be provided from other sources. If you can't live without milk, limit your intake to one or two servings per week. Buy those products that are made from grass-fed, organic, whole milk with no added sugar. Sheep, goat or A2 cow milk is preferable. Avoid all those "wholesome" dairy products such as chocolate milk, flavored milk, flavored yogurt, milk shakes or anything containing added sugar.

33

EIGHT GLASSES OF WATER A DAY

MYTH OF THE 8 X 8 RULE

We often come across statements like "Approximately 60 percent of body weight is water" ... "Our body depends on water to survive" ... "We need to drink enough water to stay optimally hydrated". These are all undeniable scientific facts. The *National Academy of Sciences* determined the *adequate intake* of water in 3.7 liters per day for men and 2.7 liters per day for women. Curious readers may ask the question, how did the Academy come up with those figures? Are the recommendations supported by some sort of scientific evidence? The short answer is no. There is no proof that men really need 3.7 liters and women 2.7 liters of water a day to remain well hydrated. Academy scientists simply took water consumption figures from U.S. survey data and they just told us we need to drink that much water. The rationale behind this theory simply implies that we need to drink a certain amount of water because we drink so much water on average. It is a totally unsupported claim.

The way scientists established *adequate water intake* values is a good example of today's typical one-size-fits-all philosophy. The body's water requirement greatly depends on the circumstances. There are many factors influencing how much water we actually need, such as our body weight, the amount of food we eat, the outside temperature, our physical activity level, our overall health and our age. Our main goal is maintaining the normal hydration level of our body. It's a scientific fact that the body's homeostasis can be maintained at a very wide range of water consumption: the more water we drink, the more water our body will excrete. The less water we drink, the less water is excreted in the form of sweat and urine.

The recommended 3.7 and 2.7 liter volumes include both the amount of water from fluids we drink, and the water contained in our food as well. As for the fluid intake, there is a common myth we often come across on health blogs and in the popular media: "Drink at least eight glasses of water a day." Professor *Heinz Valtin* at *Dartmouth Medical School* wrote a paper on this topic, trying to find the origin of the eight glasses myth.[118] The *Recommended Dietary Allowances* 1945 edition states that a suitable water allowance for adults is 2.5 liters a day including water contained in foods. Valtin hypothesizes that the myth of eight glasses came from the misinterpretation of the 1945 guidelines, by ignoring the water content of foods. Furthermore, some authors insist that caffeinated drinks don't count toward our daily water allowance. Valtin concludes there is no scientific evidence supporting the claim that we should drink at least eight glasses of water a day. As for caffeinated drinks, coffee and tea definitely count toward our daily fluid intake. For healthy individuals, thirst is the best guide for determining water intake. Besides thirst, dark-colored urine is an apparent sign that someone is dehydrated. Otherwise, you don't need to worry too much: drink water when you feel thirsty. Stop drinking when you're not thirsty anymore.

THE MYSTERY OF BOTTLED WATER

Bottled water consumption in the United States has doubled between 1999 and 2013. An average American drinks 149 liters of bottled water each year (see Figure 33.1). Although it has been around for more than a century, bottled water's success story started with the invention of the PET bottle in 1973. Since then, the bottled water industry grew into a multi-billion dollar business. It should be noted that there is a remarkable coincidence here between the revision of *adequate water intake* values and the enormous growth of the bottled water industry. I do not have evidence that the whole hydration-hoax was generated by the bottled water manufacturers, but I wouldn't be surprised if it turned out to be the case.

Under the impression of television commercials, we may assume that the bottles contain the purest form of mineral water gushing out

Bottled Water Consumption, USA

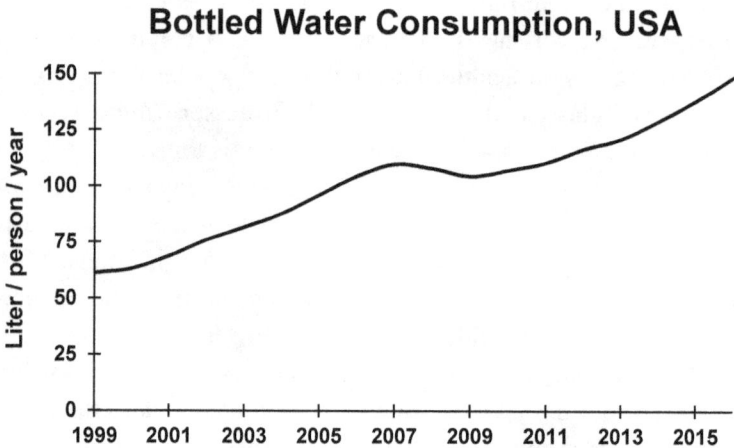

Figure 33.1. Bottled water consumption in the United States

of a rock from a picturesque mountain. Nothing is further from truth. Most of the time, it is just regular water in the bottle. The health regulations of bottled water in the U.S. are even more vague than for regular tap water. The water spends long months in the plastic bottle until it is finally consumed. Over time, plastic bottles tend to leach chemicals into water.

Massive amounts of crude oil and natural gas are required for the production of plastic bottles. Fossil fuels are used for the shipping of bottled water. The empty or half-empty bottles often end up at land-fill sites. It takes centuries for plastic to decompose. I am not an environmental activist; this is just common sense. What is the solution? If you still insist on bottled water, buy those ones in returnable glass bottles. They may be hard to find though. Don't be shy - refill water bottles with tap water or spring water. You will produce less junk and save some money that can be spent on buying some healthier food.

HAZARDOUS WASTE IN YOUR WATER

Fluoridation of drinking water supplies has been a controversial issue since the very beginning. Drinking water fluoridation was introduced in the United States in the 1950s. Proponents claim that fluorine in drinking water prevents tooth decay in children and adults. In the 1950s, several studies were published that showed a significant improvement in dental health in those communities where fluoride was added to drinking water supply. All the early studies came up with similar optimistic results. After convincing the *World Health Organization*, the fluoride mafia had launched the fluoridation program of the world's drinking water supply. Needless to say, research data proving the benefits of water fluoridation were all falsified from the beginning. The fraud was so obvious, that in 1959, a whole book was written questioning the accuracy of these clinical trials.[119] The fact of the matter is that adding fluorine to the drinking to water supply does not prevent tooth decay at all. Fluoride has a protective effect if it is applied as a *topical treatment* such as in toothpaste, otherwise it is useless. Simply swallowing fluoride does not prevent tooth decay. A U.S. study with the participation of over 39,000 school children has proved that water fluoridation has no effect on the prevalence of dental caries.[120] Fluoride is not a nutrient. Nobody has ever suffered from "fluoride deficiency". Fluoride is highly toxic and may also damage the brain. The irony of the story is that fluoride in a larger dose is not only toxic, but also damages the teeth causing a condition called *dental fluorosis*.

Readers may ask the question: if fluoride is so harmful, why is it still added to 70% of the public water supplies in the United States? The answer is simple. Water fluoridation is a huge business. Fluoride is a by-product of manufacturing plastics, ceramics, pesticides, and pharmaceuticals. Fluoride is definitely considered to be hazardous waste that is hard to get rid of. Mysteriously, instead of disposing fluoride the regular way hazardous waste should be treated, the chemical gets recycled into the drinking water supply, and some businesses even make money by doing so. In addition to these issues, there are some ethical questions as well. The U.S. *Food and Drug Administration* (FDA) classifies fluoride as a drug. Adding fluoride to drinking water is a form of medical treatment without the patient's consent.

PRACTICAL ADVICE

Don't worry too much about official dietary guidelines. If you are healthy, just drink water when you feel thirsty. Stop drinking when you're not thirsty anymore. Mineral water or spring water are the healthiest choices. If you have decent quality tap water in your area, drink tap water. Most of the time, bottled water is not any better than tap water. Contact your water supplier and make sure they don't add fluoride to the drinking water. If you buy bottled water, try to find a brand that is sold in glass bottles. Over time, plastic bottles leach chemicals into water. Avoid canned water. Aluminum cans are lined with BPA. BPA has a similar effect to *estrogens*, which are one category of female sex hormones. Try to keep plastics away from foods. A recent study showed that most plastics have estrogenic activity. [121]

Always read labels. Don't buy anything with added sugar or artificial flavor in it. Manufacturers often add sodium (salt) to water. They do it on purpose: salt makes you thirsty and they hope you will drink even more. Don't boost water sales of such food companies.

If you are a pop-addict, try to replace pops with carbonated water. Check ingredients: no sugar, artificial sweetener, acids, artificial flavor or salt. Buying a soda machine and making your own carbonated water gives you more control over what you drink. Carbonated water is not particularly harmful, but it has no health benefits either. It is slightly acidic, which may not be good for your teeth; limit the intake to one glass per day. Carbonated water contains CO^2. Carbon dioxide is the by-product of cellular metabolism. Consuming metabolic waste materials in large quantities is not likely to produce any health benefits.

34

COFFEE AND TEA

IS CAFFEINE GOOD OR BAD FOR YOU?

There is no straightforward answer to this question. Scientists have been studying the health effects of caffeine for decades, but the results are controversial. While some studies showed certain health benefits of coffee consumption, others found caffeinated beverages to be harmful. A large-scale study was done with the participation of over 400,000 men and women. Researchers examined the relationship between coffee consumption and the mortality rates from various diseases. They found that those who drink more than 6 cups of coffee a day, compared to non-drinkers, are 60% more likely to die from the most common civilization diseases including cancer, stroke, heart disease, and respiratory disease.[122] At first, we may think that there are some highly toxic materials in your cup. Fortunately, this is not the case. Statistics showed that coffee drinkers were also more likely to smoke. The harmful effects were actually caused not by coffee, but by smoking. After adjustment for smoking and other confounding factors, researchers found that the *all cause mortality* in those who drink 6 cups of coffee a day was not higher, but 10% lower compared to non-drinkers.

Coffee has a remarkable protective effect against type-2 diabetes. The top coffee drinkers had a 40% lower risk of becoming diabetic. Interestingly, decaffeinated coffee shows antidiabetic properties as well. The exact mechanism of how coffee prevents diabetes is not entirely understood. It is possible that the protective effects are caused by other ingredients than caffeine; antioxidants are good candidates. Some studies have even found that administering pure caffeine impairs insulin sensitivity.[123] Most studies agree however, that coffee, either decaf or regular, notably reduces your chances of developing diabetes.

Caffeine is therapeutically administered for the treatment of bronchial asthma, pulmonary edema, headaches, and postprandial hypotension. Coffee consumption is associated with decreased risks of neurodegenerative diseases, such as Alzheimer's disease and Parkinson's disease. On the contrary, coffee still remains a considerable risk factor for cancer (all types), based on the first paper. Another study found that high coffee intake reduces the risk of developing breast cancer in post-menopausal women by 10%, but not in younger women.[124] The risk of gastric cancer is higher and the risk of colon cancer is lower among coffee drinkers. Although the first study found a positive association between cancer risk and coffee consumption, if we examine the risks of each type of cancer separately, the results are heterogeneous. We cannot simply say that coffee consumption increases the risk of cancer in general.

From the perspective of weight loss, coffee has undeniable health benefits. Caffeine increases basal metabolic rate. It stimulates fat burning. Researchers found that administering caffeine increases fasting energy expenditure by up to 13%. Caffeine is widely used by athletes to enhance physical performance. Application of caffeine in endurance exercise increases the time to exhaustion. Administering even small amounts of caffeine results in significant improvements in the performance of swimmers, runners, and cyclists. In resistance training caffeine improves muscle strength.

Besides these benefits, caffeine has some negative health consequences as well. As mentioned earlier, caffeine may increase the risk of certain cancers. Another adverse health effect of caffeine is raising blood pressure. Coffee however contains certain natural components as well, that are capable of partially offsetting this harmful effect of caffeine. High caffeine intake is also associated with sleep disorders and anxiety symptoms.

Caffeine is the most widely used psychoactive drug in the world. Some authors claim that caffeine is addictive in nature. In order to qualify a substance as addictive, certain criteria have to be fulfilled. Caffeine meets least two of these criteria. Firstly, in absence of coffee, many individuals show the signs of *substance-specific withdrawal syndrome*. The second criterion says a "great deal of time spent in activities necessary to obtain the substance". This condition is also met, at least in North America. For example, every single day millions of Canadians religiously drive to *Tim Hortons, Starbucks* or other restaurants, patiently wait in the long line, and drive back to work once they have obtained their regular caffeine dose. In Canada, Tim Hortons alone sells 2 billion cups of coffee each year. Isn't this addiction?

Caffeine has been researched for decades, but there is no consensus among scientists whether caffeine is good or bad for your health. It is very hard to distinguish between caffeine's adverse health effects and the confounding factors accompanying coffee consumption. For example, smokers tend to drink more coffee than non-smokers do. Since caffeine and nicotine use the same pathways in the brain, habitual caffeine consumption can lead to tobacco consumption as well. This phenomenon is called *cross-sensitization*.

Caffeine is rapidly absorbed by the gastrointestinal tract. After oral intake, plasma caffeine peak is observed after between 45 minutes and 2 hours. The half-life of caffeine is the time necessary for the plasma caffeine level to fall to 50% of its initial concentration. In healthy adults, caffeine's half-life is between 2.5 to 10 hours. In children, however, the half-life of caffeine is significantly longer than that. In adult men who smoke, the half-life of caffeine is reduced by 30-50% compared to non-smokers.

In regular coffee drinkers, the direct effects of caffeine are hard to evaluate. Some researchers assume that the stimulant effects of caffeine are largely due to the reversal of withdrawal symptoms and questioning the direct effects of caffeine.

ANTIOXIDANTS IN COFFEE

Free radicals are unstable and highly reactive molecules that are capable of stealing electrons from or donating electrons to other molecules. High numbers of free radicals can damage cell components such as DNA and proteins. The process is called *oxidative stress*. Numerous diseases such as cardiovascular disease, diabetes, cancer and arthritis are associated with *oxidative stress.* Antioxidants protect us from *oxidative stress.* Raw fruits and vegetables contain considerable amounts of antioxidants. Western diets however are very low in antioxidants, because people in the industrialized countries typically consume processed food. For example, a study showed that 65% of the antioxidant intake in Norwegian adults came from coffee.[125] For those who are on a healthy, balanced diet, and their antioxidant requirements are met, coffee plays a considerably less important role in disease prevention. Either way, coffee is still a important source of antioxidants. The antioxidant content in coffee greatly depends on processing. Certain antioxidants are already present in the green bean, while others are generated during roasting. Generally, longer roasting times result in reduced amounts of antioxidants. In other words, light-medium roasts have more health benefits than dark roasts.

PRACTICAL ADVICE

Unfortunately, world's most popular coffees are the junk food's liquid equivalents. If you want to drink a healthy one, you have to make it from scratch. You need to buy light-medium roasted coffee beans and grind them shortly before brewing. Never buy pre-ground coffee. It may contain filler ingredients and other additives. Don't trust any brand name or company. Brewing methods have a great impact on the coffee's antioxidant content. Highest amounts of antioxidants are extracted from coffee by espresso and mocha machines. Paper filter coffee makers capture fewer antioxidants from coffee. Paper filters also remove oily components called diterpenes; their health effect is not entirely understood. Paper filters also leach chemicals into your coffee. This is especially true for bleached papers. According to the U.S. *Environmental Protection Agency*, white coffee papers contain dioxin, a hazardous cancer-causing chemical. If you don't already have one, you may consider investing into a good coffee maker. Those parts that are exposed to water and coffee need to be made of stainless steel or glass; the liquids shouldn't pass through other materials such as plastic or paper. Don't buy aluminum coffee makers. Stainless steel espresso or mocha coffee makers are a good choice. If you like Turkish / Arabic coffee, you don't even need any special equipment. You can easily brew your coffee in any stainless steel or glass pot without a coffee maker.

Once you have managed to solve these issues, and you are ready to make your first cup of a really healthy coffee, be careful and avoid the following pitfalls. Never serve coffee in paper, plastic or styrofoam cups. They all leach chemicals. By the way, paper cups are not just made of paper. They also have a plastic lining inside.

Never add sugar or artificial sweetener to your coffee. Although they contain virtually zero calories, artificial sweeteners trigger a similar insulin response as carbohydrates do. Avoid cow milk, unless you can buy A2 milk. For more information see *Milk and Dairy* chapter. Cream, goat and sheep milk in smaller quantities are fine.

As we have seen previously, decaffeinated coffee has similar health benefits as regular coffee. Readers may ask the question, does the process of decaffeination add any harmful chemicals to the product? Manufacturers sometimes apply chemicals to extract caffeine from coffee beans. Coffee products that are produced by applying chemical treatments definitely fall into the junk food category. However the *Swiss Water Process* is a 100% chemical free coffee decaffeination method. Decaffeinated coffee made by the *Swiss Water Process* is safe.

TEA CONSUMPTION

After water, tea is the most widely consumed beverage in Asian countries. In Asia, people have been aware of the beneficial effects of tea for hundreds of years. Green tea is made by steaming and drying fresh tea leaves to prevent fermentation. Black tea on the other hand is produced by fermentation. The third type, oolong tea is partially fermented. The antioxidant and anti-inflammatory properties of tea are attributed to its polyphenol content. Most of its polyphenols are preserved in green tea. During fermentation however, polyphenols are gradually lost. As a consequence of the processing method, black tea has a significantly lower polyphenol content than green tea. All types of tea are good for you, however green tea has the most health benefits.

Some researchers claim that coffee consumption may increase the risk of certain cancers. This is not the case with tea. The anti-cancer effects of tea polyphenols are well known. Compounds found in tea leaves inhibit the growth of human cancer cells and induce cell death in cancerous cells. Tea consumption is also associated with a lowered risk of type-2 diabetes. A Dutch study found that those who drink more than 5 cups of tea a day, are 32% less likely to develop type-2 diabetes than those who drink tea no more than once a day.[126] Regular consumption of green tea helps you lose weight and maintains your body weight. Interestingly, the weight-loss effect of tea was found to be stronger in Asians than in Caucasians. Tea consumption reduces the risk of cardiovascular disease, developing kidney stones, Parkinson's disease, and osteoporosis.

Tea is a healthier alternative to coffee. It provides all coffee's health benefits with significantly less caffeine. The caffeine content of black tea is half that of brewed coffee. Green tea contains significantly less caffeine than black tea. Don't use tea bags. Like coffee paper, they leach lots of chemicals. Buying a whole large bag of loose leaf tea from an Asian store is a good idea. Such authentic teas taste even much better than the most expensive branded varieties. Enjoy your favorite tea without adding sugar, honey or any artificial sweetener. Serve your tea in a porcelain mug or glass; paper, plastic and styrofoam cups leach harmful chemicals.

35

BEER CONSUMPTION

WHAT'S IN YOUR BEER?

From time to time, on health blogs, newspaper articles and television programs we come across authors who claim that beer drinking has several health benefits. They associate beer consumption with a reduced risk of diabetes, hearth disease, cancer, kidney stones, and osteoporosis. Some "experts" even recommend that we take our vitamin and fiber requirements with beer! I hope you don't take such claims very seriously.

Let's see how those types of studies are conducted. In *ecological studies*, researchers look for associations between the occurrence of diseases and exposure to suspected causes. For example, scientists want to prove the theory that high fat consumption causes heart disease. In this case, they can easily manufacture "massive scientific evidence" by comparing those countries with high fat consumption and high heart disease occurrence to those countries that have lower fat consumption and lower heart disease rates. After all, there are approximately 200 countries in the world, researchers can cherry pick a few of those that support their claim, just like Ancel Keys did in 1953 in his presentation. Such studies are almost useless and they don't prove anything at all. This is called *selection bias*.

In a study, beer consumption data from 47 states of the U.S. and the mortality rates of various cancers were correlated. Researchers found a strong correlation (r=0.81) between beer consumption and rectal cancer mortality in the United States.[127] Even if there were no selection bias present, the study has several limitations. There are many confounding factors such as smoking, diet, physical activity level, exposure to chemicals, etc. that can modify the risk for developing cancer. Correlation doesn't necessarily mean causal relationship. Although beer consumption may increase the risk of developing cancer, we don't know it for sure if cancer is really caused by beer itself or by other factors. The relationship between beer consumption and cancer remains controversial. Studies proving beer's harmful health effects are as plentiful as those showing its health benefits.

Despite these conflicting data, there is still sufficient scientific evidence that beer consumption is associated with many other civilization diseases. Arthritis is one of those. A case-control study was done in the UK to investigate beer's role in the development of osteoarthritis. Researchers found that those who drink more than 20 servings of beer per week are twice as likely to develop osteoarthritis in their knees or hips than those who don't drink beer at all.[128]

THE FATTENING EFFECT OF BEER

Many beer drinking nations have a common term for male abdominal obesity. The phenomenon is called "beer belly" in English, "Bierbauch" in German or "sörhas" in Hungarian. By the way, the two latter literally mean "beer belly". Everybody knows that beer is fattening. The French polymath, *Jean Anthelme Brillat-Savarin* in his famous work, *The Physiology of Taste* which was published in 1825, mentions that beer drinking nations have "huge stomachs". He also talks about Parisian beer drinkers that grew big bellies since they could not afford wine.

Besides the plentiful anecdotal evidence, there is sufficient amount of scientific research data proving beer's fattening properties. Although the process of weight gain is way more complicated than mere *calories in vs. calories out*, excess energy from beverages is a generous contributor to today's obesity epidemic. Regular beers contain 140-200 calories per 12 ounce serving. Alcohol is an energy-dense compound: each gram has 6.9 calories. Most beers contain added sugar as well. The sugar content of beer ranges from 1.5% to 6%. Little things add up. For example 5 servings of beer may contain as much as 1,000 extra calories. Along with the excess calories, cold beer may cause a very healthy appetite and you might easily end up eating more than you would consume normally.

As discussed earlier, the *calories in-calories out* model doesn't give a full, satisfactory answer to the question of *what causes obesity*. The pathogenesis of obesity is primarily regulated on a hormonal level. Insulin is the main hormone responsible for fat deposit formation. Compared to other alcoholic beverages, beer has the highest insulin-raising capacity. The *food insulin index* of beer is 20 times higher than that of gin with a 40% alcohol content.[129] The *food insulin index* is based on food samples of 1,000 kJ portions.

The exocrine part of the pancreas produces amylase enzymes. Amylase breaks down starches into sugars. Researchers found that non-alcoholic compounds in beer more than double pancreatic amylase production, while alcohol itself has no effect on pancreatic amylase.[130] Higher amylase secretion results in an increased food absorption rate and a spike in blood glucose and insulin levels. This is one of the possible explanations why beer is so fattening, especially if consumed with carbohydrate foods.

THE BIG DECEPTION

Curious readers may be wondering what beer is made of. Although beers may have quite a different appearance and taste, the basic ingredients are the same: water, malt, some sort of cereal and hops. Let's take Budweiser for example, which is America's best selling beer. According to the manufacturer's website, Budweiser is made from water, barley malt, rice and hops. Most of the time, the list of beer ingredients is very short: labels rarely show more than four components. Is that all? Well, it may have been the case 200 years ago, but it is hard to believe these claims today, when foods made from exclusively natural ingredients are very scant. Beer manufacturers don't disclose the full list of ingredients, because they don't have to. They mention just a few of the components that sound appealing to customers. The rest of the ingredients is not listed on the label. In 1990, the United States Department of Agriculture mandated that all food companies were required to list their products' ingredients on food labels. However, beer manufacturing is regulated by the U.S. Department of the Treasury, not by the FDA. The beer industry is a multi-billion dollar business. Based on 2016 data, the economic

THE SECRET OF PERMANENT WEIGHT LOSS

impact of beer in the United States was estimated to be more than $350 billion. These giant companies put tremendous pressure on governments to bend the rules, and as a result, manufacturers are not required to list beer ingredients. Food labels, as always, are very deceiving. If you look up *Nutrition Facts* data, beer doesn't look that bad at first, because the ingredient list is based on ridiculously small serving sizes, namely one ounce (see Figure 35.1). One "serving" of regular beer contains only 12 calories, which doesn't sound that much. If you do the math however, a six pack of the same beer has as many as 878 calories. Beer has no fat and no cholesterol. This statement is an indispensable part of the *Nutrition Facts* sheet and beer companies are very proud of that fact. By the way, plant foods don't contain cholesterol at all. In this day and age, people fear cholesterol more than anything else in the world. *Fat free* and *cholesterol free* are synonymous with *healthy*. Nothing is further from the truth; you can call beer whatever you want, but it's not healthy at all.

Nutrition Facts

Serving Size: 1 fl oz (29.8 g)

Amount Per Serving

Calories 12.2 Calories from Fat 0

	% Daily Value*
Total Fat 0g	0%
Trans Fat 0g	
Cholesterol 0mg	0%
Sodium 0.9mg	0%
Potassium 9.8mg 0%	
Total Carbohydrates 0.9g	0%
Dietary Fiber 0g	0%
Protein 0.1g	
Calcium	0.1%
Iron	0%
* Percent Daily Values are based on a 2000 calorie diet	

Figure 35.1. Beer nutrition facts

Enthusiastic amateurs keep on trying to solve the mystery of beer. Some web blogs claim that beer contains a whole range of harmful materials ranging from GMO corn syrup to the excretion of beavers' anal glands. My primary goal is remaining objective. Since the real ingredient list of a beer is one of the manufacturer's best kept secrets, we would be very naive if we really believed that multi-billion dollar corporations would ever release their recipes under the pressure of a few thousand web bloggers.

Instead of guessing, we could still rely on scientific literature and the opinion of independent brewing experts. Manufacturers indeed use corn syrup or other forms of added sugar to make their beer taste smoother. Although there is no direct evidence that the syrup is made from GMO corn, I am pretty sure this is the case, since 92% of the produced corn is genetically modified in the United States.[86] In 2007, unlicensed, experimental genetically-engineered rice was found in Budweiser beer.[131] Added sugars are almost as harmful as alcohol itself. We have already discussed in the previous chapters that refined carbohydrates impair insulin sensitivity. They cause continuous low-grade inflammation, which is associated with many modern-day civilization diseases such as obesity, heart disease, diabetes, and cancer. During the manufacturing process, breweries use numerous chemicals and additives that are not listed on the labels such as isinglass, gelatin, silica gel, diatomaceous earth, carrageenan, caramel, tannin, bentonite and proteolytic enzyme preparations. The fact of the matter is, some of these ingredients are carcinogenic.

In Western societies beer is the symbol of manliness. Beer drinkers should acknowledge the fact however, that their favorite beverage contains a generous amount of female hormones. The female flowers of the hop plant are used as a flavoring agent in beer. Hops contain *phytoestrogens*. The most powerful one is called *8-prenylnaringenin*. Phytoestrogens have similar effects to female sex hormones, estrogens, which are produced by the ovaries. The compound stimulates the growth of the uterus in experimental animals.[132] Due to their phytoestrogen content, hop extracts are also effective in reducing hot flashes in menopausal women. In times when hops were picked by hand, menstrual disturbances were common among female pickers.

Chronic alcoholic men often suffer from feminization symptoms such as testicular failure, enlarged breasts and a redistribution of body fat. These symptoms are explained with exposure to high levels of estrogens. Besides the phytoestrogen content, there is another source of estrogen mimics as well: beer cans are lined with BPA. A few years ago, BPA was found to be unsafe and BPA-containing baby bottles were banned in the United States.

Some of these unhealthy chemicals are dumped into our beer on a daily basis. Occasionally, even more hazardous poisons are found in beer, such as lead or arsenic. The first large-scale beer arsenic poisoning was recorded in England in 1900, affecting over 6,000 people. In the early 20th century, health regulations were vague and food science and chemistry were still in their infancy stages. The fact that arsenic can still be found in beer today sounds shocking in the high-tech 21st century. In 2013, the *American Chemical Society* announced that arsenic levels in beer sold in Germany are significantly higher than the safety limit determined by the *World Health Organization*.[133] Investigators found that arsenic was released into the beer from a filtering material used in beer production. Experts say that arsenic contamination in beer is not limited to Germany; the problem has occurred in other countries as well.

I'd like to emphasize that these were just a few examples of the known cases about the negative health effects of beer consumption published in media - only the tip of the iceberg. I purposely omitted those claims that can not be proven or have just anecdotal evidence. The only way to prevent health conditions associated with beer consumption is to not drink beer at all.

36

SALT AND SPICES

IS SALT REALLY THAT BAD?

After cholesterol, salt is considered public enemy number two. The US *National Academy of Sciences* determines the *tolerable upper intake level* of sodium in 2.3 grams per day. This is the equivalent of approximately 5.9 grams of salt, approximately a teaspoon. Here is another typical example of the *one-size-fits-all* approach. Your doctor or dietician has probably warned you already that you need to drastically cut back your salt intake. You have to do it because salt consumption causes high blood pressure that is one of the major risk factors for cardiovascular disease. The second half of the statement is correct, but how did scientists come up with the 2.3 grams per day limit of sodium intake?

The *National Academy of Sciences* in their publication[134] dedicates over 160 pages to present the scientific evidence to convince health care professionals that consuming more than 2.3 grams of sodium per day puts us at a considerably higher risk of developing cardiovascular disease. Most doctors and dieticians take *dietary reference intakes* at face value; they don't really dare to challenge those guidelines. I did what your healthcare provider most likely wouldn't ever do: I went through the scientific literature, did additional research, and applied some critical thinking as well. It turned out that the 2.3 gram limit was chosen arbitrarily. There is no such scientific evidence that consuming more than 2.3 grams of sodium per day would increase the risk of cardiovascular disease.

It may sound shocking to mainstream scientists that the 1945 edition of the *Recommended Dietary Allowances* states that the normal daily intake of salt is 10-15 grams (3.9-5.9 grams of sodium). Those doing heavy labor or working in hot climates may even consume 20-

30 grams of salt daily (7.9-11.8 grams of sodium). On the contrary, the 1977 *Dietary Goals For The United States* aims to cut back salt consumption to 3 grams (1.18 grams of sodium). After World War II, when refrigeration began to displace salt's traditional role in food preservation, salt consumption in the U.S. dropped dramatically. During the 1950s and 60s, salt intake was gradually cut down to half of pre-war quantities. In the same period, the mortality rates from coronary heart disease rose higher than ever before in the history of mankind. A drastic reduction in our salt consumption obviously did not decrease coronary heart disease mortality rates at all. Following government recommendations, very often the dietary measures' health effect is just the opposite of the desired outcome.

"A half-truth is even more dangerous than a lie. A lie, you can detect at some stage, but half a truth is sure to mislead you for long." The quote is from the Indian anesthesiologist and writer, *Anurag Shourie*. Medical journals and books are full of half truths. Scientific research is directly or indirectly funded by the multi-billion dollar pharmaceutical and food industries. Those papers that don't support the sponsor's idea never get published. Even the published results are very controversial.

Let's take a quick look at how the whole salt hysteria started. In the *cholesterol* chapter, we read about Ancel Keys' "doctored" diagram. In 1953, Keys cherry-picked six countries and drew a graph showing a nearly linear relationship between fat consumption and heart disease death rates. Figure 36.1 shows a similar diagram. The *x axis* depicts the urinary sodium excretion (the indirect measure of sodium intake) and the *y axis* indicates the systolic blood pressure of the subjects. The chart is based on data from the *Intersalt Study*, published in 1988.[135] Although the design and methodology of Keys' presentation and the *Intersalt Study* are quite different, there is a common feature. The authors cherry-picked the subjects to prove the truth of their theory. Scientists call that *selection bias*. The graph shows a linear relationship between salt consumption and blood pressure. The more salt you eat, the higher your blood pressure gets. Are you sure? Take a look at the four points marked with circle. They are not even close to the rest of the data points. Statisticians call them

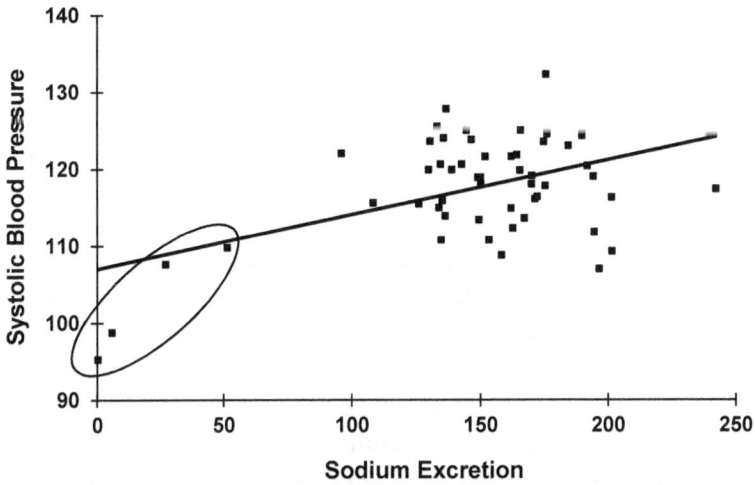

Figure 36.1. Sodium excretion and systolic blood pressure based on data from 52 locations

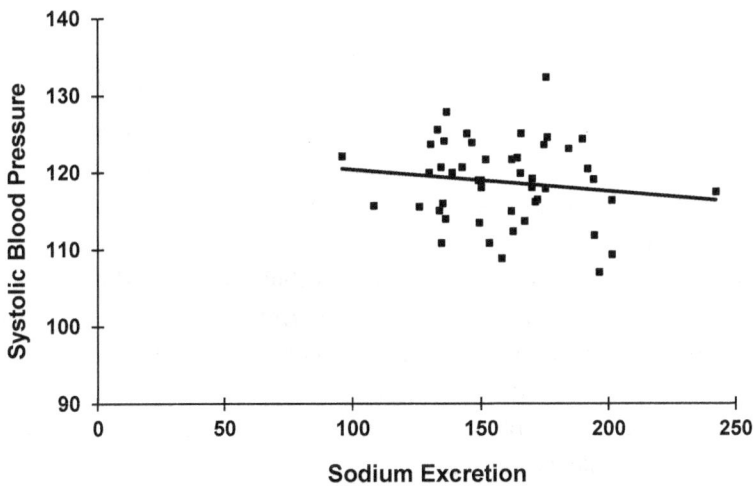

Figure 36.2. Sodium excretion and systolic blood pressure based on data from 48 locations

outliers. Those data were taken from four tribal communities in Kenya, Papua New Guinea; the Xingu and Yanomamo Indians of Brazil. Their salt consumption is next to nothing. Such data are completely irrelevant. Hunter-gatherer tribal communities can not be compared to the United States or Japan. Surprisingly, if we omit the data collected from indigenous people, the trendline goes just the opposite direction: an increase in salt consumption slightly decreases blood pressure, see Figure 36.2. It should be noted that the second correlation is not statistically significant (p=0.3). The *Intersalt Study* falls into the category of observational studies. By their nature, these types of studies don't provide very strong scientific evidence. However, clinical trials give the most rigorous evidence of causality.

The British Medical Journal published a review of 34 randomized clinical trials.[136] Researchers examined the effect of reduced salt consumption (on average, a 4.4 gram daily reduction) on blood pressure with the participation of 3,230 individuals. Lower salt intake had just a minor beneficial effect by slightly reducing blood pressure. On average, systolic blood pressure decreased by 5.4 mm Hg and diastolic blood pressure by 2.8 mm Hg. That's all. Other studies found that salt intake below a certain threshold even lowers blood pressure. The *Dietary Reference Intakes* book of the *National Academy of Sciences* has several endnotes. Out of curiosity, I followed a few of the references to check out how the Academy came up with the infamous 2.3-gram sodium limit. The fact of the matter is that there is no such scientific evidence to justify the 2.3-gram rule. The results of the relevant studies show just the opposite of what we expected. For example, one of the cited studies found that a low-salt diet not only has zero health benefits but is even harmful; it slightly increases blood pressure and drastically raises plasma renin activity and aldosterone levels.[137] The study found that a 4.6-gram daily sodium intake results in the lowest blood pressure. This amount is twice as high what we were told by the Academy.

Public health media keeps on telling us the half truth: salt consumption raises blood pressure. Does it? There is no "yes" or "no" answer to the question. It greatly depends on the individual and the circumstances. The same study suggests that 60% of the population is not sensitive to sodium; even if they consume high amounts of salt, they can maintain a normal blood pressure. For example, the Japanese use more salt and still suffer less from hypertension and live longer than people in most countries. In healthy individuals, high salt intake has no adverse health effects since excess sodium is excreted in urine. A low-salt diet increases renin activity and aldosterone levels. Both renin and aldosterone cause hypertension and they play a key role in the regulation of blood pressure. Low sodium intake adversely affects insulin resistance, blood lipids, and increases cardiovascular disease risk. Considering both the risks and health benefits, a low-salt diet is not recommended for healthy young individuals. Based on the presented scientific evidence, the optimal blood pressure, renin and aldosterone levels are associated with a moderate sodium intake ranging from 2.3 to 4.6 grams per day. This is the equivalent of 6 to 12 grams of salt consumption, one or two teaspoons of table salt. You don't need to count grams, but avoid excessively salty foods, for example fish products preserved by salting. On the other hand elderly people who suffer from hypertension, and African Americans are in the high risk category. Their salt intake should be reduced.

THE MYSTERY OF REFINED SALT

Table salt is substantially different from the salt that comes out of the mine. While raw salt is a little bit chunky and has a grayish or brownish color, refined salt is bright white with uniform crystals. Two things happen to raw salt before it gets packaged: valuable minerals are extracted and chemicals are added to it. Have you ever wondered why those "impurities" are removed from salt? Are they harmful? Not at all. In order to maximize profit, the minerals are sold separately at a higher price. Natural salt contains considerable amounts of calcium, magnesium, potassium and many other elements. For example, by switching to unrefined salt, we will cover 100% of our daily magnesium and 12% of our calcium requirement. Refined salt, on the other hand is stripped of its mineral content. In order to have nice uniform crystals and to get the salt to come out of the shaker smoothly, we need to add some chemicals to the salt. The food industry calls them *anticaking agents.* Some of these compounds are harmless, while others are really nasty ones. Salt additives often contain aluminum, that is linked to dementia. The other ominous chemical is called *potassium ferrocyanide.* As the name implies, it contains the deadly *cyanide,* C≡N group. Thanks to the strong chemical bondage between the *cyanide* group and the iron however, the toxicity of this compound is not very high. An average consumer eats only 1/200,000 of his lethal dose daily. What about long-term exposure? The answer is, we don't know. Nobody has ever studied the health effects of lifelong *potassium ferrocyanide* consumption. I'd just like to point out the attitude of the big food companies: if you don't die from their products within 30 days, they don't really care. It should be noted, the same C≡N (*cyanide*) group can be found in *amygdalin,* that was successfully used in the treatment of terminally ill cancer patients who literally had nothing to lose, until FDA outlawed *amygdalin.* On the other hand, the FDA approved *potassium ferrocyanide* for everyday use by *healthy* individuals just to let table salt flow more smoothly. The FDA's double standard rules may seriously affect the health of millions.

IODIZED SALT

Iodine is essential for good health. The thyroid gland uses iodine to produce thyroid hormones. Thyroid hormones increase the basal metabolic rate, affect protein synthesis, growth, neural maturation, and have many other vital functions as well. Besides the thyroid functions, iodine is also an antioxidant, stimulates the immune system, and prevents cancer, especially in the breasts, ovaries and prostate gland.

There is a common myth that unrefined sea salt contains all our iodine needs. Unfortunately, this is not true. The iodine content of unrefined salt makes up just a little fraction of our daily iodine requirement. As you probably noticed, food labels don't show the product's iodine content. Have you ever wondered why? Iodine is an extremely volatile chemical element. If exposed to air, it evaporates easily, even at room temperature. Although it is present everywhere, the concentration of iodine greatly varies from place to place. In highest quantities, iodine can be found in the body of marine animals and plants. In coastal areas, the soil's iodine content is high. Plant foods grown in such places are rich in iodine. Similarly, the meat of animals fed with iodine-rich food has high iodine content. In land-locked regions however, the locally produced food is low in iodine. For example, a century ago, the areas around the Great Lakes in Canada and the United States were called the "goiter belt" because of the high prevalence of severe iodine deficiency. Those people who live in coastal areas, eat local food only, including a lot of seafood, probably meet their iodine requirements. For the rest of us however, in order to avoid deficiency we need additional iodine sources.

Over the course of the past century, governments worldwide made extraordinary efforts to promote the use of iodized salt as a primary measure to prevent goiter, the most obvious sign of iodine deficiency. Although goiter itself is a very rare disorder in the United States, it doesn't necessarily mean that every single American gets a sufficient amount of dietary iodine. In some countries, including the U.S., food manufacturers don't use iodized salt. As a result of increasing sales of processed foods, people get significantly less iodine than a few decades earlier. Even those who regularly use iodized salt can suffer from iodine deficiency. Iodine is extremely volatile. Salt should be kept in an airtight container. Once the package is open, iodine starts to sublime immediately. An experiment was done with various salt samples, to find out how long it takes to lose the iodine content of the salt after opening the package.[138] The results were shocking. If the relative humidity level is 90%, the whole iodine content will be gone within a month. Even if the salt is stored in dry places, half of the iodine is lost within a couple of days.

I am not encouraging anybody to purchase food that contain chemical additives. All our nutrient requirements should be supplied from natural ingredients. In the case of iodized salt however, we can make an exemption. In case your requirements cannot be supplied by naturally occurring iodine in your food, iodized salt should be added to your diet. Like always, read labels. Make sure no other ingredients are added other than potassium iodide; no anticaking agents and other chemicals.

Seaweed is a very rich natural source of iodine and many other valuable nutrients including vitamin B12. For example, our daily iodine requirement can be satisfied by 4 grams of dried *nori*. Seaweed consumption is an indispensable part of Japanese cuisine. A hundred years ago, before the introduction of Western food, iodine deficiency was non-existent in Japan, although salt was not iodized. On the other hand, in the "goiter belt" of the United States 26-70% of children had clinically apparent goiter, before the 1920s.

There are some environmental and nutritional factors that impair the bioavailability of iodine. Bromine is the main adversary of iodine. Although it is banned in Canada and the European Union, bromated flour is still widely used in the United States. Brominated vegetable oil in canned beverages is another dietary source of bromine. We are surrounded by bromines that can be found in fire retardants, plastics, pesticides and household chemicals. Bromine may be added to the water of swimming pools as a chlorine alternative. Smoking is another risk factor for iodine deficiency. Some plant foods contain glucosinolates, which when consumed in high quantities, may interfere with thyroid gland functions. Such plants include cabbage, broccoli, cauliflower, kohlrabi and kale. Otherwise, these foods are very healthy and they shouldn't be neglected. When eating these vegetables, we need to intake some extra iodine.

SPICES AND HERBS

Spices and herbs have been considered as a powerful remedy for various human disorders since ancient times. Some plants have a remarkable blood glucose-lowering effect such as cardamom, onions, garlic, fenugreek, turmeric, cumin, ginger, mustard, curry leaves, coriander, ginseng, cinnamon and nigella. These plants promote weight loss and have numerous other positive health effects as well.

For healthy individuals, being on a bland diet is not recommended. The health benefits of spices and herbs is inexhaustible. Some plants show anti-inflammatory properties, while others help to lower cholesterol levels and regulate blood pressure. Spices contain valuable minerals, vitamins and antioxidants. Unlike in the case of salt, you can use as much as you want of all varieties of spices.

Always read labels. Never buy those products that contain sugar, food additives or have any ingredients other than the spice itself. Consume spices as close as possible to their natural state with minimal processing. For example, don't use ground pepper. Buy whole peppercorns and grind them directly on your meal as needed. Cook with fresh garlic instead of garlic powder. Processed spices and herbs lose a lot of their valuable nutrients and you can never be sure what other ingredients they may contain. Fresh herbs also taste much better.

37

THE VITAMIN HOAX

THE RISE OF THE JUNK FOOD INDUSTRY

We may be under the impression that junk food was invented by McDonald's and KFC in the 1950s. The fact of the matter is that the history of the junk food industry can be traced back much earlier. Hamburgers, hot dogs, French fries, sugar-sweetened beverages, chocolate, ice cream and candies already existed in the 19th century. Junk food however was not part of the everyday diet. The consumption of such foods was limited to special occasions such as county fairs, circuses, and sporting events. The origin of junk food itself however goes back even further. In the United States, the adulteration of food started over two hundred years ago. With the advancement of technology, mills could process grain fast, cheaply, minimizing labor by using new methods. As a result of the industrial revolution, inexpensive flour flooded markets throughout the United States. However, consumers have paid a very high price for the cheap flour: by using the new technology, the bran and germ of the wheat kernels got removed. These removed parts are the ones that contain the most valuable nutrients such as proteins, fibers, minerals and vitamins. An American preacher, *Sylvester Graham* launched America's first food protest movement. Graham pointed out that white flour coming from the new mills was unhealthy and began advocating the consumption of locally produced whole grain wheat flour. Unfortunately, people didn't listen to Reverend Graham and over the 19th century, whole grain flour got gradually displaced with the cheap white flour. The worst thing however, was still yet to come. Sugar, before its mass production, was only available to the elite classes who could afford it. As production increased and prices dropped, the precious commodity became an everyday item. During the past two hundred years the average American's sugar intake rose nine fold. The over-consumption of highly refined carbohydrates was accompanied by an unhealthy lifestyle, which paved the road to the epidemic of modern-day diseases such as obesity, diabetes, heart disease, arthritis, cancer and many others.

THE DISCOVERY OF VITAMINS

Until the end of the 19th century, only four essential nutrients were known: proteins, carbohydrates, fats, and minerals. Scientists believed that all diseases are caused by infectious organisms. Even non-communicable diseases such as scurvy, beriberi, rickets, and pellagra were considered to be infections. The *vitamin theory* originated from the French chemist, *Jean Baptiste Dumas*, who discovered that milk contains certain indefinite substances employed in the sustenance of life. Even the smallest and most insignificant traces of these compounds seemed to be not only efficacious, but even indispensable. The term "vitamine" was invented by the Polish biochemist *Casimir Funk*, who found that vitamins B1, B2, C, and D were necessary for human health. In his 1912 paper, Funk pointed out that many diseases previously considered to be infectious are actually caused by vitamin deficiency. Casimir Funk's work lead to the discovery of 13 vitamins over the course of the next decades.

THE SCAM OF VITAMIN SUPPLEMENTS

Half of the US population uses dietary supplements. One third of Americans regularly take vitamin pills. Readers may ask the question: why are vitamins so popular? *"Nomen est omen "* is an old Latin saying: "The name speaks for itself". The never before seen popularity of vitamin supplements today can be explained not only by professional marketing techniques deployed by big pharmaceutical companies, but partially also by the name itself (*vita* means life, *amine* is an organic compound). I would call *Casimir Funk* a real genius for inventing the word *vitamin*. Imagine if vitamins wouldn't be called vitamins, but had a less fancy and marketable name, for example *essential organic compound* (EOC). Would EOCs sell as much as vitamins do? I don't think so. Thanks to Casimir Funk, the vitamin industry grossed $12.8 billion in the United States in 2017. This amount of money would be enough to buy 85 million tons of wheat that could feed 450 million people for a whole year. As per FAO, the number of undernourished people is over 800 million worldwide. In other words, the amount Americans spend on vitamin supplements alone would cover half of the cost to totally eradicate hunger from the face of the earth.

Do vitamin supplements work at all? The short answer is no. Unless you suffer from a certain vitamin deficiency, they are absolutely useless. For example if you have pellagra, vitamin B_3 can save your life. Otherwise taking vitamin B_3 tablets is absolutely unnecessary. The supplement industry takes the advantage of the credulity of the people. Do you really think that you can stay healthy simply by regular consumption of vitamin supplements while eating junk food and living a sedentary lifestyle?

Do you remember *Ancel Keys*? I would call him the father of cholesterol hysteria. Thanks to Keys, the medical research derailed for decades by ignoring the fattening effect of refined carbohydrates and blaming the coronary heart disease epidemic on dietary fat. Nevertheless, Ancel Keys made one remarkable discovery: in 1942, he experimentally proved that vitamin supplements are useless.[139] Ironically, the world accepted Keys' bad advice and rejected the good advice.

The vitamin-hero, *Linus Pauling* came up with a strange theory in the 1960s. He claimed that a whole range of diseases can be prevented by taking mega-doses of vitamin supplements. Pauling suggested that vitamin C can prevent not only the common cold, but also heart disease and cancer. Although Linus Pauling was the only person ever to win two unshared Nobel prizes, there is no scientific evidence that these conditions can be prevented by taking large doses of vitamin supplements. The fact of the matter is, that some studies found vitamin supplements to be not only useless, but rather even harmful.

In 2018, the *Journal of the American College of Cardiology* published a meta-analysis of 179 clinical trials[140]. Researchers analyzed the cardioprotective effect of vitamins A, B_1, B_2, B_3, B_6, B_9, C, D, E, multivitamin and mineral supplements. The study found no evidence that any of these vitamins would reduce the risk of cardiac events. Surprisingly, vitamin B_9 turned out to be a serious risk factor, increasing the chance of coronary heart disease by 47% and stroke mortality by 85%.

Nobel prize-winner *Linus Pauling* claimed that "75% of all cancer can be prevented and cured by vitamin C alone". Other vitaminists use B vitamins to combat cancer. Unfortunately none of these work. A Norwegian study showed that patients who received a B_9 and B_{12} vitamin treatment were 21% more likely to be diagnosed with cancer.[141] The vitamin prevention of cancer and heart disease fails for the same reason: vitamins and antioxidants interfere with free radicals, which are generally considered to be harmful because they may damage the DNA and proteins. However, free radicals also play an important role in *apoptosis*, the programmed cell death. The elimination of free radicals leads to an uncontrollable cell growth, as seen in cancerous cells and in smooth muscle cells in the wall of atherosclerotic arteries.

Representatives of the pharmaceutical industry argue that our foods don't contain enough vitamins and minerals; to preserve our health we need take dietary supplements regularly. I'd like you to notice, this is just a sales technique. There is overwhelming scientific evidence that in most cases vitamin supplements have no health benefits at all; sometimes they are even harmful. A healthy diet contains all the necessary nutrients and there is no need of taking artificial vitamins or any other dietary supplements.

38

CALCIUM CRAZE

HOW MUCH CALCIUM DO WE REALLY NEED?

"Research suggests that half of Americans aren't getting enough calcium." … "Calcium is essential for building and maintaining strong bones." … "Calcium helps muscles work and helps nerves carry messages between the brain and other parts of the body."

When watching television, reading newspapers or surfing the internet, we come across slogans like these on a daily basis. The creativity of the marketing experts hired by pharmaceutical companies is amazing. Obviously, those schemes work: in the United States nearly half of adults and 70 percent of older women regularly take calcium supplements. Due to the pushy sales techniques of the pharmaceutical companies, selling crushed limestone and calcium citrate tablets to otherwise healthy people grew into a multi-billion dollar business.

Calcium is the fifth most frequently occurring element in our body. Calcium is indispensable. I am not disputing the physiological role of calcium. However, there are three important questions need to be answered: How much calcium do we actually need? Do dietary calcium supplements really prevent osteoporosis and bone fractures? What are their possible risks and long-term side effects?

The *Recommended Dietary Allowances* (RDA) of calcium for adults is 1,000-1,200 mg/day, depending on age. Let's take a quick look how these recommendations were established. The governments of the United States and Canada requested *the Institute of Medicine* (IOM) to carry out a comprehensive study to determine the RDA values for calcium and vitamin D. The *Institute of Medicine* completed the study and established the *Recommended Dietary Allowances* for calcium and vitamin D. Their guidelines are considered the industry standard in North America. In 2011, the *National Academy of*

Sciences published a 1,133-page book on the study with detailed explanations.[142]

Before we go into technical details, let me mention an important fact: an obvious conflict of interest that the Academy failed to disclose. The *Institute of Medicine* (now called *National Academy of Medicine*) both *directly* and *indirectly* receives substantial amounts of funding from the pharmaceutical industry.

For example, the 2015 annual report of the *Institute of Medicine* listed all the major pharmaceutical companies as their sponsors with a contribution amount of $1 million to $5 million such as *Pfizer, Merck, GlaxoSmithKline, AstraZeneca Pharmaceuticals* and *Eli Lilly and Company*. They also listed *Novartis Pharmaceuticals* and *Sanofi* with an unspecified amount. These are the companies who make your everyday medications. In many cases, pharmaceutical companies don't fund research directly. They do it through their "philanthropic" and "charitable" organizations such as *Wellcome Trust* or *The Rockefeller Foundation*. I just scratched the surface. The deeper you dig, the more evidence you will find that our whole healthcare system is entirely controlled by the pharmaceutical industry. Big Pharma doesn't want you to be healthy. They try to put you on life-long medication instead.

Let's start with our first question: How much calcium do we actually need? The correct answer is, nobody knows exactly. Over the years, researchers developed a few methods to determine our calcium requirements based on examining bone mineral density and bone fracture rates or calcium balance studies. In adults, our goal is maintaining a neutral calcium balance. In other words, to avoid bone loss, calcium intake should be the same as the amount of calcium leaving the body. *Hunt and Johnson* did a series of nineteen feeding studies conducted in a metabolic unit. Researchers examined the subjects' calcium intake and the amount of calcium excreted in the form of urine and feces.[143] The study found that a neutral calcium balance is achieved at a calcium intake of 741 mg per day. The *Institute of Medicine* took the 741 mg data, rounded it up, added a safety margin and established their 1,200 mg recommendation for women. That's a significant difference: 1,200 vs 741 mg. There is another key statement in the original report that calcium proponents never mention: "...calcium balance was highly resistant to a change in calcium intake... " The authors found that the calcium homeostasis can be maintained in a wide range of calcium intake of 415-1,740 mg/day without suffering calcium losses.

Just for curiosity's sake, I looked up how much calcium intake was recommended a century ago. The 1928 book *Nutrition* by *Walter H. Eddy* established the adult male's calcium requirement in 450 mg per day, with a safety margin of 680 mg. This is pretty close to *Hunt and Johnson's* recent findings. Readers may think that today, by using the latest technology, researchers can estimate our calcium requirements more precisely than a hundred years ago. I have to object. Calcium balance studies don't require any high-tech equip-ment. All we need to do is to measure the amount of calcium entering the body and the amount of the excreted calcium. The same principle applies today as a century ago.

The short answer to our second question is that taking calcium supplements hardly prevents osteoporosis and won't reduce the risk of bone fractures. Scientists have been studying dietary calcium's bone fracture preventive effect for decades. The *Women's Health Initiative Trial* was one of the largest studies ever done. With the participation of over 36,000 postmenopausal women, researchers examined the effects of dietary calcium and vitamin D_3 supple-ments.[144] Taking calcium tablets for years showed virtually zero health benefits. To be precise, the hip bone's mineral density increased by one percent over the course of nine years, however the risk of bone fractures remained the same in both the calcium and the placebo groups. That was not all. Calcium supplementation not only turned out to be absolutely useless, but also had a harmful side effect. Those subjects in the calcium group were more likely to develop kidney stones.

SUMMARY

We can conclude by saying that dietary calcium supplements don't prevent osteoporosis and bone fractures. The best way to preserve your bone health is adopting a healthy diet and remaining physically active. Regular physical exercise has numerous health benefits: it increases the body's insulin sensitivity, burns calories, improves muscle tone, and strengthens bones.

In order to preserve your bones, avoid excessive amounts of animal protein that can be found in dairy and meat products. Commercials try to convince us that milk is the healthiest food in the world. Nothing is further from truth. The negative health effects of commercially produced milk have been already discussed in the *Milk and Dairy* chapter of this book. Official recommendations for dairy consumption are unrealistic. For example, if you want to cover all your calcium requirements from milk alone, you need to drink a liter every single day. This is a lot of milk. Although milk is rich in calcium, its casein content substantially outweighs the supposed health benefits. In addition to that, the body's calcium balance is negatively affected by the increased acid load caused by the intake of animal proteins. As a result, more calcium will be excreted from the bones. Interestingly, those countries with the highest milk consumption also have the highest rates of osteoporosis and bone fractures. For example, the Swedish consume 12 times more dairy products than the Chinese, and the hip fracture rate is 8 times higher in Sweden than in China.[145]Based on the scientific evidence previously discussed in this chapter, milk consumption and dietary calcium supplements don't prevent osteoporosis and bone fractures.

39

NEGATIVE CALORIES

THE BENEFITS OF VINEGAR

Vinegar has been very popular since ancient times for both cooking and medical purposes. The word *vinegar* comes from Old French, meaning sour wine. Vinegar is very easy to make at home. Wine at room temperature in the presence of oxygen is fermented by bacteria and the alcohol content will be gradually converted into acetic acid, the main ingredient of vinegar. Not only wine, but all fermentable fruits and grains can be turned into vinegar. There are many different types of vinegar. Fruit, balsamic, cane and grain vinegars are the most widely used varieties.

The medical use of vinegar dates back millennia. Vinegar has remarkable antibacterial properties. Hippocrates 2400 years ago recommended vinegar for the treatment of sores and ulcers. Vinegar also helps fight obesity and prevents a whole range of diseases associated with being overweight such as hypertension, hyperglycemia and hypercholesterolemia. The health effects of vinegar were studied on 175 obese Japanese subjects. By the end of the 12-week treatment period, those who consumed 30 ml vinegar a day, on average lost 2 kg of body weight. Abdominal fat areas were noticeably reduced, and the cholesterol, blood sugar and blood pressure values significantly improved.[146]

Vinegar is a very powerful weight-loss tool and should be added to your everyday diet. As a practical advice, when shopping for vinegar, you don't need to buy the most expensive and fanciest product. The simple white vinegar will do the job for you just like an organic apple cider vinegar. Always read labels. Watch for carbohydrate / sugar content. Manufacturers usually add sugar, to make vinegar taste smoother. Some varieties may contain as much as 25% sugar.

Needless to say, products like that fall into the junk food category. Buy those products with a total carbohydrate content of less than one percent.

DIETARY FIBER

Dietary fiber has numerous health benefits, including reducing the risk of developing some cancers, hyperlipidemia, hypertension, coronary heart disease and type-2 diabetes. Fibers slow down the absorption rate of carbohydrates and reduce the post-meal insulin response. As a result of lower insulin levels, less energy will be deposited in fat cells. You can find more information about dietary fiber in the *Man's Best Friend* chapter of this book.

IODINE

Iodine is essential for good health. The thyroid gland uses iodine to produce thyroid hormones. Thyroid hormones help you burn fat by increasing the *basal metabolic rate*. In developed countries, iodized salt is the main dietary source of iodine. Although health authorities recommend the use of iodized salt, I don't agree with this practice for two reasons. First, iodized salt contains other chemicals besides iodine as well. Second, after opening the package, the iodine content of the salt evaporates within weeks, making iodized salt useless. Use unrefined salt instead. It also tastes much better. The iodine requirement of our body can be entirely covered naturally from dried *nori* seaweed.

For more information visit the author's website. Scan the code on the right with your device.

40

THE CASE AGAINST MICROWAVES

THE MICROWAVE HOAX

Microwave ovens heat foods quickly and conveniently. Most households and restaurants use them every day and our modern world would be hard to imagine without microwave ovens. They make our lives easier by warming up leftover food without burning it in the pan. You can also thaw your frozen dinner in a microwave oven within minutes. Although most of the time, microwave ovens are used just to warm up food, you can cook in them as well. Many microwave cookbooks and recipes are available online. However, for some reason, meats prepared in a microwave oven don't taste as good as those cooked traditionally. There is a common belief that microwaves cook from the inside out. This myth however turned out to be incorrect. Some people – including myself – say that microwave prepared meats taste like the sole of a shoe. Nevertheless, either used for cooking or just for warming up food, microwave ovens are indispensable these days.

Have you ever heard that microwaves are harmful? There are tons of websites suggesting that you throw out your microwave oven, claiming that escaping radiation from your oven may damage your health, and that microwaved food causes cancer. Internet celebrity *Joseph Mercola*, one of the most famous proponents of alternative medicine wrote an article on the harmful effects of microwaves entitled *How Your Microwave Oven Damages Your Health In Multiple Ways?* People naturally fear radiation coming from electronic devices. I googled these keywords *"microwave"* and *"cancer"*. The search returned over 31 million results. It should be noted however, that internet search engines don't belong to the smartest forms of artificial intelligence. Very often, search engines bring up irrelevant things or show the same results repeatedly. Nevertheless, even if we accept only a tiny little fraction of the 31 million hits, we still definitely have a serious issue here that should be further investigated. Direct exposure to a certain level of microwave radiation is dangerous. This is a scientific fact. What about indirect exposure? What happens if our food gets irradiated? Some experts claim that you don't need to be exposed to microwaves directly, you can even get cancer by eating microwaved food. Let's see where these allegations come from. I did some in-depth research and I found that virtually every single internet article on the harmful effects of microwaves is based on information that can be traced back to four sources.

The first author is the mysterious *William P. Kopp* of Portland, Oregon. I don't believe in the existence of either *Santa Claus* or *William P. Kopp.* If you google the name *William Kopp*, the results include a famous poker player, a family physician, two politicians: one from the 19th and one from the 20th century. Our friend is none of them. Under the name of *William P. Kopp*, an article entitled *Effects of Microwaves on Humans* was published in *The Journal of Natural Science* in 1998. At first, it seems that there is nothing wrong with the journal. It has a prestigious-sounding name just like the *National Geographic Magazine.* I regret to say that *The Journal of Natural Science* is not a real scientific magazine. I would definitely put that paper in the pseudoscience category. In addition to that, there are other, real scientific journals that have very similar names. This is quite deceiving. The ominous report which is also available on the internet, has a subtitle "FORENSIC RESEARCH DOCUMENT T061-7R10/10-77F05; RELEASE PRIORITY: CLASS 1 R001a". At first glance, the article seems like an abstract of a scientific research paper. Although the vocabulary and style of the whole document suggest that the author is familiar with the terminology of life sciences, the paper contains numerous incorrect facts and statements. Such claims include that the microwave oven was invented by the Nazis and that the Soviet Union banned microwave ovens in 1976. The latter is a very common myth deliberately propagated by anti-microwave activists. The logic behind the gossip is that microwaves are so harmful that even the evil communist regime outlawed them, but the microwave lobby in the Western world intentionally retains the evidence against microwaves. Of course, such rumors are not true. I personally own a photograph of a 1980 microwave oven made in the USSR.

Here comes the tricky part: *Kopp* claims that microwaves create "d-nitrosodiethanolamine (a well-known cancer-causing agent)". I did some research. Three major chemical search engines: *ChemSpider, PubChem* and *ChEBI* don't show any evidence that the aforementioned compound exists at all. The closest matches are *N-nitrosodiethanolamine* and *nitrosodiethanolamine,* which are indeed cancer-causing chemicals but they are not exactly the same compound that *Kopp* claims. We should keep in mind that the paper was written in 1998 during the internet's infancy years. In those days, everything wasn't available online. It would have taken a trip to a university library to verify the correct name of the compound, so the author just relied on his imagination instead.

If you look up *d-nitrosodiethanolamine* in a non-scientific search engine e.g. google, which has 6,900 matches for the questionable molecule, most results refer to websites that simply copied Kopp's article. Many pages even literally quoted the phrase "a well-known cancer-causing agent" from the original article. That was not all. At the end of the *Kopp* article, the editor even inserted a foot note that the powerful microwave lobby forced *William Kopp* to change his name and to disappear. At this point we have no more doubt that it is just a hoax. Ironically, the made-up story was so successful, that somebody even falsified it. This one-page "research document" is even more widely available on the internet than the original one. The falsified version of the fake story had numerous errors and inconsistencies. For example, the alleged Oregon researcher used British English and the zeroes on the file number are replaced with capital Os. In addition to that, the poor wording of the whole document clearly suggested that the author was not a scientist.

The third hoax is the most absurd of all. Google "microwaved water - see what it does to plants". The anonymous document showed photos of two plants that allegedly were watered with either purified water or microwaved water. By day nine basically there was nothing left from the plant that was treated with microwaved water. Did the plant dye from the irradiated water? No. If you zoom in on the picture, it is clearly visible that the leaves were simply cut off.

Swiss engineer *Hans Ulrich Hertel* conducted an experiment back in 1991. Eight subjects in a health resort were studied for a period of two months. Participants were put on a diet consisting of traditionally cooked and microwaved food items. Hertel found that the consumption of microwaved food significantly affects the blood cell counts and cholesterol levels. However, the experiment could never be reproduced by others and the results were not published in peer-reviewed scientific journals. In other words, Hertel's findings can not be accepted as scientific evidence.

IS MICROWAVED FOOD SAFE?

The short answer is, most likely it is safe, but we don't know for sure. Just because health authorities declare microwaving safe, it doesn't necessarily mean there are no long-term negative health effects. On the other hand, I think there are many things in our lives that are definitely proven to be harmful such as refined carbohydrates, the habit of constant grazing, overeating or a sedentary lifestyle. We shouldn't worry too much about the unproven theory of the negative health effects of microwaved food.

In my opinion, microwave ovens should be treated the same way as plastics: use them if only there are no any better options. I recommend microwave ovens for warming up leftover food only, but not for cooking or thawing frozen food. Take your food from the freezer half a day before you need it and let it sit at room temperature. Microwave it slightly right before you eat.

PART

FIVE

HOW TO LOSE WEIGHT PERMANENTLY

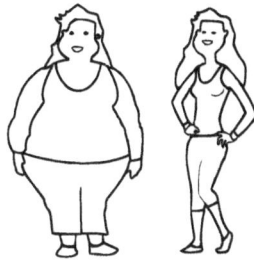

41

THE FIVE PILLARS OF HEALTH

CIVILIZATION DISEASES

Heart disease, cancer, respiratory diseases, stroke, Alzheimer's disease, diabetes are the six deadliest diseases, claiming 1,726,000 lives in the United States each year.[147] What is common in these health conditions? They are all lifestyle diseases, as they can be directly linked to the way people live their lives. Diabetes, heart disease, stroke, cancer, and dementia have been known since ancient times, however they were extremely rare. For example, Homer's *Odyssey*, which was written approximately 2,800 years ago, mentioned that King Laertes, the father of Odysseus suffered from dementia. According to the story, Laertes wore rags and lived in a goat shed. He couldn't even recognize his own son, Odysseus, when he returned from the Trojan War. Diabetes was also well known by ancient Greeks. *Aretaeus* describes the disease as "melting down of the flesh and limbs into urine". Stroke was first described by Hippocrates more than 2,400 years ago. Researchers found signs of cancer and coronary heart disease in Egyptian mummies. The Bible mentioned that King Eglon was an extremely obese man. The king was assassinated with a dagger. He was so fat that when he was stabbed in his belly, the fat closed upon the blade and the grip of the weapon. Turkish researchers did a study of the health conditions of 36 emperors of the Ottoman dynasty who reigned between 1258 and 1926. Over 80% of the sultans were obese; more than half had non-fatal cardiovascular events and one third suffered from metabolic syndrome.[148] I am using these examples to illustrate that there is nothing new about lifestyle diseases. Although these conditions have been in existence since ancient times, they affected the ruling class only; normal people rarely suffered from such diseases until 200 years ago.

Since the end of the 18th century, the industrial revolution brought major changes, not only in production and the economy but in the society as well. People started migrating to nearby cities from rural areas and gave up their traditional lifestyle. New technologies made it possible to refine both grains and sugar very efficiently. Healthy whole grain flour got gradually displaced by cheap white flour. Sugar, before its mass production, was only available to the elite classes who could afford it. As production increased and prices dropped, the precious commodity became an everyday item. During the past two hundred years, the average American's sugar intake rose nine fold. The increasing consumption of highly refined carbohydrates accompanied with a physically less and less active lifestyle paved the road to the epidemic of many modern-day diseases. Parallel with the advancement of technology and urbanization, such diseases became more and more common. For example, Napoleon's physician, *Stanislas Tanchou* used to say that "Cancer, like insanity increases with civilization". By the early 20th century, lifestyle diseases were no longer limited to the wealthy people only. The new worldwide epidemic of obesity, heart disease and cancer was on the rise. An interesting fact is that *William Osler* in his 1921 book, *The Principles and Practice of Medicine* still calls heart disease rare; he estimates only *one case a year* per hospital, even in big metropolitan areas. In contrast today, heart disease is the number one killer in industrialized countries.

Over the past 100 years, the prevalence rates of various lifestyle diseases have been rising rapidly. Remarkably, during World War I and World War II, such diseases temporarily recessed, due to food shortages. Later, once the war was over and food became abundant, diseases were on the rise again.

Through these examples, my intention was to illustrate that most of our modern-day civilization diseases are the direct result of our unhealthy lifestyle. Although lifestyle diseases are typically preventable, our governments, scientists and healthcare providers don't really make sufficient efforts to prevent such disorders. Public policies for dealing with those issues are limited to the treatment of the symptoms alone, leaving the underlying causes of the diseases them-selves untouched. Why is this happening?

In the United States, healthcare is a three trillion (million times million) dollar industry and food sales gross over five trillion dollars each year. Most experts agree on the point that the whole healthcare system is extremely inefficient and very corrupted. Scientific research is very often funded by the food and pharmaceutical indus-tries. Medical schools are controlled by the pharmaceutical lobby. By relying on the principles of our corrupted mainstream science, healthcare professionals give bad advice and we just get sicker and heavier each year. Big Pharma doesn't want you to be healthy, they are perfectly fine with the present situation. The profit-driven healthcare system is not really interested in the prevention of these avoidable diseases. Big Pharma wants to keep you on lifelong medi-cation instead. Suppressing the symptoms with expensive drugs instead of eliminating the underlying cause of the diseases is the typical approach of today's Western medicine.

HOW TO STAY HEALTHY

Did you know that during the 20th century, civilization diseases claimed more lives than all other diseases, wars, violent events and dictatorships combined, including World War I, World War II, geno-cides, civil wars, man-made famines and communism?

It doesn't have to be that way. By changing our lifestyle, we can significantly reduce the risk of the most common civilization diseases such as obesity, type-2 diabetes, heart disease, stroke, cancer, demen-tia, osteoporosis, arthritis, asthma, depression, and others as well. Many of these medical conditions have been known for millennia, but they were extremely rare. If we don't have a time machine and go back in time in order to stay healthy, what other options are available for us?

Dan Buettner, working with the National Geographic Society, spotted five regions around the world where people live the longest. These places have the highest number of 100-year-olds and many people grow old without diseases like cancer, obesity, diabetes or heart disease. The healthiest and longest-living people in the world can be found in Sardinia, Italy; Icaria, Greece; Okinawa, Japan; Costa Rica and among the Seventh Day Adventist communities in California. These regions are known as *Blue Zones*.[149] Although the language, the culture and the customs of these places are quite different, the lifestyles of these people show many similarities. The world's healthiest people live a physically active life. In order to stay in good shape, *Blue Zones* people don't need to go to the gym. They do long-lasting, low-intensity physical work instead, such as gardening and household chores that keep them busy all the day. In place of driving, they walk a lot. The healthiest and longest-living people live a purposeful life. They put their families first and actively participate in community events.

Despite the different customs, the diet of the *Blue Zones* people is very similar. Their food is predominantly plant-based, consisting of mainly grains and vegetables. Meat is eaten only once or twice a week. Milk and dairy intake is limited. There is no added sugar in their everyday diet. Sweets are reserved for special occasions.

THE FIVE PILLARS OF HEALTH

Eat Healthy Food

There is an ancient saying, that is attributed to *Hippocrates*, the father of medicine: "Let food be thy medicine and medicine be thy food". There is two thousand years of wisdom in this sentence. Unfortunately, prevention is often neglected in our profit-oriented, modern, Western medicine that heavily relies on drugs, surgery and radiation to suppress the symptoms (signs of illness), instead of eliminating the underlying causes of the diseases themselves. The vast majority of our modern-day lifestyle diseases can be prevented. That's exactly why they are called *lifestyle diseases*, because they are the direct result of the individual's way of living. I'll go even further. A healthy diet not only prevents many diseases, but also is often capable of reversing serious, life-threatening conditions that are considered to be progressive and irreversible.

Here are two concrete examples. *Dr. Caldwell Esselstyn*, a prominent heart surgeon came up with a revolutionary new idea. He started treating heart disease with dietary measures. In 1985, Dr. Esselstyn initiated a small study.[150] Severely ill patients with coronary artery disease were put on a whole-food, plant-based diet. After 12 years, 17 out of the adherent 18 patients had no cardiac events at all. Twelve patients had a follow up angiogram. The examination showed a remarkable disease reversal in four of them. The rest of the group showed some moderate improvement, but most importantly no future cardiac events occurred. These positive results were confirmed by a second, larger study with the participation of 198 patients. Dr. Esselstyn calls heart disease "a toothless paper tiger, that need never ever exist, and if it does exist, it need never ever progress".

Mainstream medicine considers type-2 diabetes as an incurable, progressive disease that gets worse and worse over time. When first diagnosed, many people with type-2 diabetes can keep their blood glucose at a normal level simply by oral medication. Over time, as insulin resistance gets worse and worse, diabetes cannot be controlled by oral medication alone. The patient will end up on a small amount of insulin, then on more and more insulin. As a matter of fact, the disease will just get worse and worse over time.

However, Canadian nephrologist, *Dr. Jason Fung* has a different opinion. The doctor calls diabetes a dietary disease that needs a dietary treatment. Dr. Fung, the founder of *Intensive Dietary Management Program* is specialized in the treatment of obese individuals with type-2 diabetes. By implementing strict dietary measures and lifestyle changes, Dr. Fung's patients experienced a significant improvement in their fasting plasma glucose and *HbA1C* levels. In many cases, diabetes was completely cured and after completing the program, patients were off medication.

These two examples have demonstrated that healthy food plays a central role not only in disease prevention, but often is even capable of defeating serious, life-threatening disorders. A healthy diet is the most important pillar of our good health. Whether we become healthy or sick is determined by our food in the first place.

Be Physically Active
Regular physical exercise is an indispensable part of healthy living. Exercising helps you maintain your cardiovascular health; it strengthens your bones and muscles, reduces the risk of some

cancers, increases insulin sensitivity, improves your sleep, and relieves stress. Most lifestyle diseases are closely linked to a sedentary lifestyle. The healthiest and longest-living people in the world regularly participate in all sorts of physical activities. You don't need to be an iron man or run marathons to preserve your health. If you have a sedentary lifestyle, half an hour of medium-intensity exercise five or six times a week will be good enough. Strenuous physical exercise longer than one hour a day has no additional health benefits.

Get Adequate Sleep

Sleep plays an important role in the preservation of your physical health. Not getting enough sleep does more than just make you feel tired. Sleep deprivation increases the risk of a whole range of diseases including high blood pressure, heart disease, stroke, diabetes and obesity. Adults need at least 7-8 hours of sleep a day.

Reduce your Stress Level

Lifestyle diseases are directly or indirectly linked to our stressful, modern-day life. Long-term stress exposure not only makes you sick but also causes weight gain. The stress hormone *cortisol* is one of the major regulators of our fat metabolism. Elevated cortisol levels stimulate fat deposition, especially in the abdominal area of our body. Slow down. Avoid stressful situations if possible. Make sure you get an adequate amount of sleep. Exercise regularly. Working out is the most efficient form of stress relief.

Live a Purposeful Life

All the *Blue Zones* people have something to live for beyond just work. Finding a purpose for your life may add years to it. Canadian researchers after analyzing statistical data of over seven thousand individuals found that living a purposeful life is one of the most important predictors of longevity.[151]

42

WHY ARE DIETS USELESS?

MYRIAD OF DIETS

Diet books are very popular these days. I did a quick search on *Amazon*: the keyword "diet" returned over 60,000 hits. Diet programs are sold under various names. Even though each one looks slightly different, all of them have the same common elements. Every single diet book contains a "hook". Some diets promise a quick weight loss, while others claim that you will lose weight effortlessly, or you can eat as much as you want. However, the most important common feature of every single diet is that they all fail in the long run. There is no exception.

THE TAXONOMY OF FAD DIETS

Fad diet is a well-known and widely used term to describe diets that obviously don't work in the long run. There are different types of fad diets. The same way that biologists put animals into various classes such as amphibians, reptiles, birds etc., similarly, can we also differentiate between three main categories of weight-loss diets. There are *dangerous*, *hoax* and *temporary weight-loss* diets. By the beginning of the 21st century, obesity had become an uncontrollable worldwide epidemic. Day by day, millions of dieters fight their hopeless battle with obesity. Although the vast majority of diets is useless and harmless, some strange weight-loss techniques can even put dieters at a considerable risk.

DANGEROUS DIETS

The creativity of self-proclaimed diet "experts" is endless. The most absurd diet I ever heard of is swallowing tapeworm eggs. Tapeworms are parasites of domestic animals, for example sheep and cattle. After grazing animals ingest worm-contaminated food, worm eggs hatch in the intestines and through the blood vessels the larvae spread throughout the host's body. When raw or undercooked meat of an infected animal is eaten, humans may become infected with tape worms. Over time, the worms can grow up to 10 meters long in the human digestive system and they may live up to 25 years. It is like a horror movie, resembling the 1979 film *Alien*, but this one is true. Proponents of the tapeworm diet argue that you will lose weight because your worm eats up the nutrients directly from your guts. Let me ask a question: at what price? Nurturing a real 30-foot monster in your body?

HOAX DIETS

A big portion of the available diets fall into this category. Hoax diets are not particularly dangerous to your health, but they don't help you lose weight either. The authors either come up with an unproven pseudo-scientific statement or take a scientific fact out of the original context. Let me mention a few examples of hoax diets: *Blood Type Diet, Macrobiotics Diet, Juice Fasting, The Moon Diet Plan* or *Cookie Diet*. *Dr. Sanford Siegal* came up with a brilliant business idea in 1975: the doctor encouraged his patients to snack on cookies between meals. Despite the lack of scientific evidence and the astronomically high prices (hundreds of dollars for one month's cookie supply) the diet-cookies sold so well that Siegal managed to build up a multi-million dollar diet empire on selling weight-loss cookies.

"Eating chocolate every day can help you lose weight." Have you heard this claim before? In 2015, a ludicrous team of journalists in Germany fooled the whole world for a short period of time. They published a scientific research paper based on a fake clinical trial showing that chocolate consumption causes weight loss. The story made headline news in more than 20 countries and half a dozen languages. The experiment was a good example of human credulity.

TEMPORARY WEIGHT-LOSS DIETS

Diets that don't fall into the first and second category, may cause you lose weight in the short run. Such weight-loss techniques however are very deceiving. You may easily go through a 10-pound weight loss even in one single week! For example, novice dieters may experience such weight-loss phenomenon during the first week of the Atkins diet. Although the scale may go down drastically, the missing pounds mostly come from fluid loss, some glycogen, and a reduced amount of food passing through the digestive tract, not from the fat deposits.

Let's say you chose a diet program that seems to be working, and after long months of suffering, you finally manage to lose 20 pounds of body fat. You are very happy with your weight loss. After you have achieved your goal, you decide to stop torturing yourself and go back to your regular way of living. What do you think will happen? Do you believe that you will be able to keep the pounds off for the rest of your life? The sad reality is that immediately after you quit dieting, pounds will just slowly keep on coming back. It's only a question of months, probably a year and you will end up weighing the same, perhaps even more than before you started dieting, despite your heroic efforts. Then, you have to start a new diet program one more time. After long months of suffering you will lose weight again, which won't last long either, and so on. The phenomenon is called *yoyo dieting*. It seems like there is an invisible mechanism that controls your body weight in the long run, just like the thermostat regulates the temperature of your house. It make no difference, what protocol you follow, virtually, every single diet is destined to fail. They all work the same way and you can not achieve a permanent weight loss by simply dieting.

Dr. Atkins' *Diet Revolution* book sold more than 15 million copies, making it one of the best-selling diet books ever written. Since 1972, it is estimated that 20 million people worldwide went on the Atkins diet. Where are the long-term results? For example, we have never heard of people who went on Atkins diet 10 years ago, lost 50 pounds, and have kept the weight off.

William Banting's *Letter on Corpulence* made it to the world's first and very popular diet book. Although the book itself was extremely successful, Banting was not so successful in loosing weight himself and keeping the weight off permanently. Do you know what was similar in the stories of Dr. Atkins and William Banting? Both weight-loss experts died obese. How is it possible? Either their regimen didn't work for the authors or they simply weren't able to stay on their own diet for a longer period of time.

BEWARE OF FALSE TEACHERS

Here are my practical tips on how to spot those false teachers. When evaluating a weight-loss program, make sure that the author
-was once obese
-achieved a substantial weight loss
-stayed thin for the rest of his life
If any of these three criteria are not met, be extra careful. There is a very good chance that the whole diet is just a scam.

WHY ARE DIETS DESTINED TO FAIL?

We have seen so far that dieting is useless. By taking advantage of the credulity of people, from time to time, clever businessmen come up with absurd ideas such as *The Moon Diet Plan*, the *Cookie Diet* or the *Chocolate Diet*. Apart from such bogus schemes, the next category is the group of the "temporary weight-loss diets". The whole concept reminds me the *temporary grasses*. Years ago, a company was selling grass seed. They had a very impressive commercial showing a perfectly green, healthy lawn that could survive even underneath the snow. However, there was a serious issue, concerning the product itself: buyers were never told that they are purchasing the seeds of an annual grass species, that would die off at the end of the season. Going on a diet is just as useless as sowing temporary grass seeds in your backyard: none of these two will produce permanent results. Even if you pick a diet that works in the short run, and successfully manage to get rid of your extra pounds, your weight loss will just be temporary. Immediately after you finish your diet program, the pounds will just slowly keep on coming back. It's only a question of months or a year, and you will end up weighing the same, despite your extraordinary efforts. This phenomenon is called the *thermostat effect*. Your body desperately defends the preset weight, regulated by your invisible inner "weight thermostat". Every single diet works the same way. Why are all diets destined to fail?

There are two difficulties here that you have to overcome. First, you need to lose a certain amount of weight. There are many weight-loss techniques that may work for you in the short run. However, weight loss is just the easy part. Keeping the weight off permanently, without torturing yourself for the rest of your life is the real challenge. You simply cannot be on a diet forever.

Obesity is a typical lifestyle disease. It is a direct result of our unhealthy way of living. Obesity was extremely rare until 200 years ago and it is still not present in today's primitive societies. In order to lose weight and also keep the pounds off permanently, you need to completely change your whole lifestyle. As mentioned earlier, obesity is a lifestyle disease and it can not be treated with dieting alone. Dieting just suppresses the symptoms of the disease, but does not affect the underlying causes of obesity itself. Dieting is like treating a bad tooth with painkillers without seeing a dentist. You need to do much more than just simply dieting: you have to completely change your unhealthy lifestyle. By doing that, you will not only lose weight, but you will also keep the weight off permanently and will also be much healthier. In the *Building Blocks of Weight Loss* chapter you can find a practical guide on how to achieve these goals.

43

DETERMINE YOUR GOALS

HUMAN LONGEVITY AND HEALTH

As we saw earlier, people in *Sardinia, Icaria, Okinawa, Costa Rica* and the *Seventh Day Adventist*s in California live significantly longer than the rest of us. These places have the highest number of 100-year-olds and many people who grow old without diseases like cancer, obesity, diabetes, dementia or heart disease. These people don't need to make New Year's resolutions to lose weight. They don't read diet books. People in *Blue Zones* don't go to the gym to stay in good shape. They just remain fit and healthy until almost the very end of their lives.

Most of us are not so privileged to live on the sunny coasts of a Mediterranean or Pacific Ocean island. The health benefits of a mild climate, lots of sunshine and a quiet lifestyle in a natural environment are undeniable. However, even without a tropical island you can still build your own *Health Zone* right there where you live. The secret of longevity, the secret of health and the secret of permanent weight loss are not really secrets. The information on how to achieve these goals has been known for millennia.

There is a very common myth. Popular science media often gives you the impression that these days, thanks to the advancement of science and technology and our modern health care system, the *maximum human lifespan* is significantly higher than ever in the history of mankind. From time to time, scientific papers are published claiming that the human life expectancy has almost doubled over the course of the past two hundred years. It's a fact that during the industrial revolution the life expectancy of the British working class in the crowded cities was very low due to poor nutrition, hygiene, work and housing conditions. However, even two centuries ago, men didn't typically die in their 30s or 40s, as some authors suggest. Although the *life expectancy at birth* was significantly shorter than today, the *maximum human lifespan* hasn't changed much.

What about antiquity? Let's take Greece for example. Did ancient Greeks typically die in their 30s or 40s? Not really. Greek scientists analyzed the life span of 83 individuals who lived in the Golden Age of ancient Greece between the 5th and 4th century B.C. The subjects were all renowned men living at that time, whose data of birth and death have been chronicled with certainty. Researchers found the average life span of these ancient Greek man to be 71.3 years.[152] This is pretty close to the life expectancy of men who live now, 2500 years later.

Psalm 90 of the *Bible*, which was written by *Moses* in 1300 B.C., says that the number of years of a human life is seventy or eighty. This is twice as much as the life expectancy was in England during the industrial revolution. We can conclude that the human lifespan has been nearly constant for more than 3300 years. Even in ancient times, those who were not slaves of others, lived in peace, had enough food, and did not suffer from extreme poverty were expected to live as long as today's people.

SET YOUR GOALS AND MAKE THEM HAPPEN

Throughout the previous chapters of this book, you probably noticed that I don't really believe in dieting. Diets are just a temporary fix and they don't really offer a permanent solution for your weight problem. Obesity is a very complex disorder. The most widely accepted *calories in-calories out* model grossly oversimplifies the causes of obesity. In *The Formula for Weight Loss* chapter, we saw that the question of *What causes obesity?* is much more complex than previously thought. Calories, nutrients, fasting, hormones, genetics, your lifestyle and even the duration of obesity have a significant impact on your body weight. Caloric intake is just one of the several *terms* of this very complex equation. By just cutting back on your calories, you won't address the underlying causes of obesity, and the pounds will gradually come back sooner or later. Authors of regular weight-loss diets typically focus on reducing caloric intake only but they don't see the whole picture. That's why such methods simply fail in the long run. Instead of useless dieting you need to do something else. You have to make radical changes in your way of living.

First, determine your goals. Most people want to be lean, healthy and live long. These are realistic expectations. Obesity is associated with a wide range of diseases and health conditions. By reaching your ideal body weight and living a physically active life, you will significantly reduce the risk of developing numerous modern-day civilization diseases such as type-2 diabetes, heart disease, stroke, arthritis and many others. Achieving a healthy weight goes far beyond aesthetics. We need to look at obesity differently. The results of the latest research show that body fat is much more than just an energy storage medium. As a matter of fact, fat tissue is the largest endocrine gland of our body. It produces hormones, and other chemical signaling molecules as well, so-called *cytokines*. Some of these cytokines have adverse health effects. They keep the body in the state of a continuous, low-grade inflammation. Most of the diseases of our modern-day life such as obesity, type-2 diabetes, cardiovascular disease, stroke, arthritis and cancer are associated with continuous, low-grade inflammation. If you eliminate the underlying cause of those life-threatening diseases, you will live a longer, healthier life. We have never heard of obese 100 year olds.

Think big. Let's say you used to be very lean when you were younger and you want to weigh the same as back in your high school years. Nothing is impossible. It's totally up to you. Here is my personal testimony. I, the author of this book, was obese for very long, for a quarter of a century. During those years, I tried a few conventional techniques in order to lose weight: I drastically cut back my food intake, exercised every single day for nine years and used weight-loss pills as well. None of the traditional methods worked for me. All of these previous attempts failed and either had only a minimal weight-loss effect, or the weight just came back after a few months. Back in 2016, I finally came to the conclusion that it was nearly impossible to loose weight and also keep the weight off for a long period of time using conventional methods. I went through the medical literature diligently looking for the answer to the great question of *Why do all diets fail in the long run*? (*The Formula for Weight Loss* chapter explains the basic principles of a successful weight-loss program). I realized that permanent weight loss can not be achieved simply by dieting. Obesity is a lifestyle disease and we need to completely change our lifestyle in order to combat obesity. Based on my new model, after 25 years of obesity, I finally managed to lose 55 pounds in total. Now, I weigh the same as back in high school (this is not even the graduation weight but that one measured in grade 10). My BMI went down from 31 to 21. I feel 25 years younger. I can run again. Climbing a hill is not a problem. The best part still has to come: Not only have I lost 55 pounds, but I was also able to keep the same exact weight since 2016. This is the point where regular diets fail. Losing a certain amount of pounds is one thing, but keeping the weight afterwards is the biggest challenge. Keep on reading. In the following chapters, I will explain why regular diets don't work in the long run and what steps you need to take to achieve a permanent weight loss. Regardless if you want to go back to the same weight as when you were back in high school, or just want to lose some extra pounds, the following chapters will guide you through those steps to achieve your goals.

44

BUILDING BLOCKS OF WEIGHT LOSS

WHY WERE WE GIVEN WRONG ADVICE?

Have you ever wondered why there are any obese doctors? For example, *Dr. Robert Atkins*, the father of the famous Atkins diet was one of them. Although Dr. Atkins authored one of the best selling diet books ever written, people who personally knew the famous diet doctor, described him as "obese".

Even though extreme cases of obesity rarely occur among physicians, two thirds of them still fall into the overweight category, just like the general population. Doctors treat all sorts of diseases; they are the experts of the physiology of the human body. How is it then possible that physicians are just as obese as the rest of us?

In order to further investigate the question, let's see how mainstream medicine treats obesity today. What kind of advice are we given? Here are a few examples of the most common strategies we use to combat obesity: eat less, exercise more. Avoid fat, eat more fruits and vegetables. Count calories. Drink several glasses of milk every day. Snack between meals. Eat six meals a day. Take multivitamins, mineral supplements. You have the perfect recipe for disaster. People are just getting more and more obese every year.

Although most healthcare professionals never question the official guidelines, there are promising signs. Some physicians have realized that conventional methods have failed and we need to re-consider the way obesity is treated. In 2018, 717 Canadian physicians signed a petition to the Minister of Health, demanding to review the official dietary guidelines in Canada. Current recommendations are based on U.S. dietary guidelines that date back more than 40 years. In 1977, the *Nutrition Committee of the United States Senate* formulated a paper entitled *Dietary Goals for the United States*. For the first time in U.S. history, the government told the citizens that they could improve their health by reducing the fat and increasing carbohydrate consumption in their diets. This infamous paper had more impact on our health than any other dietary guidelines ever published. Since 1977, virtually every single country adopted the US recommandations that basically haven't changed during the past four decades.

Ironically, the introduction of the new dietary guidelines coincided with the beginning of the largest obesity epidemic in human history. We were given bad advice and scientific research was derailed for decades. We have already discussed in the previous chapters that the fattening effect of carbohydrates had been well known for two centuries. However, during the 1960s and 70s, despite the lack of scientific evidence and because of political reasons, cardiovascular disease was blamed on fat consumption and people were encouraged to eat more carbohydrates. As our carbohydrate intake had increased, so did our body mass index and the prevalence rate of many modern-day diseases.

In addition to putting the whole world on a low-fat diet, let's see what else is wrong with mainstream medicine's approach towards the treatment of obesity. According to the *World Health Organization*'s definition: "The fundamental cause of obesity and overweight is an energy imbalance between calories consumed and calories expended." In the *Calories In, Calories out* chapter we discussed that calorie counting doesn't work in the long run. The *calories in - calories out* model grossly oversimplifies the human metabolism. In addition to calories, there are other factors as well that have a significant impact on your body weight, such as nutrients, fasting, hormones, genetics, lifestyle, and even the duration of obesity. The *calories in - calories out* model focuses on only one of the potential causes of obesity.

In addition to these issues, there is another bad habit we have developed over the course of the last few decades. It is the obsession with constant "grazing". In the second half of the 20th century, with the invention of snack food, our eating habits changed radically. By adding three snacks to our regular breakfast, lunch and dinner, the

251

pattern of our insulin production changed drastically. As a result, we are in a continuously high insulin state, that causes insulin resistance over time, and also greatly increases the risk of becoming obese. There are more details in the *What to Eat vs. When to Eat* chapter.

Chapters 8 to 15 give a very detailed answer to our most important question: *What causes obesity?* All my statements are backed by scientific evidence and endnotes with references to scientific literature. In order to get a better understanding of the actual cause of obesity, I recommend reviewing Chapter 15, *The Formula for Weight Loss*, if you haven't done so yet.

THE BUILDING BLOCKS OF WEIGHT LOSS

In the following chapters, we will see how you can build up your own *Health Zone*. I will give you my personal guidance and lots of practical advice on how to reach your ideal body weight, keep the weight off permanently, and prevent many modern-day civilization diseases. The building blocks of the program are broken down into the following modules:

- *The Eating Window*
- *The Right Food*
- *Physical Activity*
- *Other Weight-Loss Factors*

45

THE EATING WINDOW

THE IMPORTANCE OF TIMING

In the *What to Eat vs. When to Eat* chapter I have mentioned that the fattening effect of foods depends not only on the food itself, but it is also greatly influenced by the time of the day your meal is consumed. In other words, the question of *when to eat* is almost as important as *what to eat*. In this chapter, we will introduce various timing techniques to help you to allocate your food intake throughout the day in order to minimize their fattening effect. We will cover the following topics: How many meals should we eat in a day? When should we have the first and the last meals of the day? What is intermittent fasting? What is the main difference between the eating pattern of the *early bird* and the *night owl* types?

THE SIX MEALS A DAY MYTH

A very common advice given by doctors and dieticians is that we should eat six times a day. Instead of our regular breakfast, lunch and dinner we are often told having six small meals throughout the day. Another version of the six-meal plan is adding three snacks between our regular meals. Proponents of frequent eating argue that constant "grazing" helps you lose weight. Some experts think that frequent eating increases energy expenditure due to the thermogenic effect of food. Their second argument is that eating six small portions instead of three larger meals suppresses hunger and increases satiety. Although the idea of having six meals a day is very popular among healthcare professionals, it completely lacks any scientific evidence. Let's examine where this very common myth comes from. The whole concept is based on animal experiments. More than half a century ago, researchers found that rats eating 6 to 8 meals a day are leaner compared to those animals eating once or twice a day. Basically that's all. Animal experiments were followed by several human studies that had very controversial results. Most of these experiments had a very small number of participants, typically 6 to 20 people. Instead of precise clinical trials, many of the studies were based on health surveys or self-reported data, both of which are not very reliable methods. We can conclude then, that there is no scientific evidence for that claim that having 6 meals a day really helps you lose weight.

THE EARLIER THE BETTER

There is an old proverb that says, "Eat breakfast like a king, lunch like a prince, and dinner like a pauper". Although the adage is not entirely correct, there is a lot wisdom in it. The saying points out the importance of timing: the bulk of our caloric intake should be allocated between the morning hours and noon. Let's take a closer look at why. For example, if you eat two identical meals, one served in the morning and one in the evening, they don't have the same fattening effects. As many would find out, the same food consumed in the evening causes more weight gain than if eaten in the morning. The body's insulin sensitivity is significantly higher in the morning hours than later in the day. Researchers found that the same meal results in a 75% higher increase in blood sugar levels if consumed in the evening rather than in the morning.[49] The last meal of the day should be taken at the earliest possible time and one should completely avoid eating late at night.

FASTING AND WEIGHT LOSS

As we discussed previously, increasing meal frequency, e.g. having six meals vs. three meals a day, is definitely not going to help you to lose weight. Let's take a quick look at the physiology of the human body to see why constant eating leads to obesity. The consumption of carbohydrate meals increases blood sugar levels. High blood glucose levels are followed by an insulin rush. Insulin is the main regulator of fat storage in our body. Elevated insulin levels divert nutrients into your fat deposits instead of burning up the energy in lean tissues. However, researchers found that not only carbohydrates, but proteins increase blood insulin levels as well.

The more often you eat, the more energy will be deposited as body fat. On the other hand, while fasting, just the opposite thing happens. The body gradually uses up its own energy deposits instead of putting nutrients into storage. When exogenous glucose (the sugar from the food) runs out, glycogen from the liver and muscles will be converted into glucose. Once glycogen reserves are depleted, typically within 16 to 20 hours, body fat becomes the primary source of energy. The longer the fast is, the more fat you burn. It's so simple. The idea of losing weight while constantly "grazing" is a nonsense. The concept of nonstop eating interferes with the basic physiological principles of the human body.

It should be noted that traditionally we used to eat three meals a day, back in those times when we were still lean. In the second half of the 20th century however, with the invention of snack food, we were encouraged to eat 3 extra meals between our regular breakfast, lunch and dinner. As snacking became a regular habit in our fathers' days, the upcoming new generations grew heavier and heavier. Today, when two or three additional meals are part of our diet, obesity has become a worldwide epidemic. You can read more about this topic in *chapter 13* entitled *What to Eat vs. When to Eat,* where I discussed the physiology of fasting in more detail, supported with references to scientific literature.

THE EATING WINDOW

As we saw before, during eating periods, your body stores the unused extra calories in the form of glycogen and body fat. On the contrary, when you are fasting, the body gradually uses up the stored nutrients to keep you moving. Therefore, while you are in the feeding period, you are continuously gaining weight. On the other hand, while you are fasting, you are constantly losing weight. It makes perfect sense. In other words, in order to lose weight, we need to narrow down the eating window as small as we can. Don't have unrealistic expectations, however. The *one meal a day diet* is getting more and more followers these days. As the name suggests, those who are on this protocol, eat only once a day. Remember, every single diet fails in the long run. No exception. Let's see, what's wrong with this approach. Having just one meal a day, for weight-loss purposes is nearly ideal, I am not disputing that part. However, are you ready to commit to eating only once a day for the rest of your life? Seriously? How long would you be able to follow such an excruciating diet? Sooner or later you would quit for sure.

We have seen so far, that a very narrow eating window is an extremely powerful weight-loss tool, but the protocol is hard to follow for an extended period of time. We should keep in mind we are not dieting. All diets fail in the long run. We are changing our lifestyle instead, in order to lose weight, keep the weight off, and stay healthy for life. We have to choose a long-term, sustainable plan. I recommend an 8-hour eating window. For example, you eat breakfast at 8 AM, lunch at noon and dinner at 4 PM. By following this plan, your eating period is 8 hours a day, while the fasting period is 16 hours. If you are on this regimen, for most of the day you are in a fasting state, dominated by low insulin levels. As a result, instead of building up fat deposits, the calories will be burned in the lean tissues of the body.

Let's compare this plan to the conventional six-meals-a-day-constant-"grazing"-eating pattern. If you follow doctors' recommendations, as a result of non-stop eating, you will be in a continuously high insulin state all day long until the second half of the night. As a consequence of the constantly high insulin levels, instead of burning up calories in the muscles, the energy will be deposited as body fat. Detailed explanations can be found in the *What to Eat vs. When to Eat chapter*. For those who can not keep the 8-hour eating window, it can be extended to ten hours. However, under no circumstances should be the feeding period longer than twelve hours a day.

EARLY BIRD 🐦 VS. NIGHT OWL 🦉 TYPES

We are all different. Some people perform better during the morning hours, while others are more active in the evening. To a certain extent, we are all capable of changing our daily routines. However, turning a real evening-type person into a morning person is not an easy task and for some individuals going through such changes is nearly impossible. For example, the early bird schedule may not be suitable for those who work long hours or who are more active during the evening hours. There are some people who are not hungry in the morning at all, but simply can not fall asleep with an empty stomach. If this applies to you, and after many attempts you weren't able to adopt the early-bird-eating-pattern, do what's natural for you: just follow the *night owl*'s schedule instead of becoming an *early bird*.

We should keep in mind however, even the same food has a much more fattening effect if it is consumed in the late night hours rather than in the morning. In other words, the earlier you have your meal, the more you can eat without getting obese. To overcome the problem, I have a solution for those who simply can not adopt an early bird lifestyle. If you are a night owl type, follow this schedule: Eat the first meal of the day at noon and the last one at 8 pm. You can still customize your eating pattern the way it is convenient for you, but the time period between the first and the last meal of the day shouldn't be longer than 8-10 hours. Don't forget, while you are fasting, your body is burning calories.

INTERMITTENT FASTING

Intermittent fasting is getting more and more followers these days. As people recognize that conventional diets simply don't work in the long run, many dieters are switching to intermittent fasting instead of pointless *weight cycling* techniques. Intermittent fasting is an extremely powerful tool in weight management and is the centerpiece of both weight-loss and weight-maintenance regimens.

Intermittent fasting is so efficient that it is even capable of reversing type-2 diabetes, which was called an incurable, progressive disease by the *American Diabetes Association*. The common feature of obesity and type-2 diabetes is that both disorders are linked to insulin resistance. Fasting greatly improves the body's insulin sensitivity. Based on the same principle, a hundred years ago, in the pre-insulin era, *Elliot Joslin* successfully treated over 1,300 diabetic patients with intermittent fasting. Although Joslin's method targeted the underlying cause of the disease, his protocol is not used these days. For today's profit-oriented, Western medicine, it is more convenient to suppress the symptoms with expensive drugs, regardless of the consequences.

Let's see how intermittent fasting works. The whole concept is based on alternating cycles of fasting periods and regular eating days. On fasting days no food is allowed, but there is no limit on non-caloric fluid intake. The typical length of a fasting period is 24 hours. Depending on the subject, longer fasting periods (36 to 48 hours) can also be incorporated. The longer the fasting day, the more efficiently fat burning goes. Fasting that lasts longer than 48 hours is not recommended. Even a 24-hour fasting protocol can greatly improve the body's insulin sensitivity, and in most individuals results in a sustainable, long-lasting, weight-loss effect. In addition to increasing insulin sensitivity, intermittent fasting also leads to a negative energy balance. While you fast, your body has no other, external energy sources and has to burn your own body fat. In addition to these health benefits, intermittent fasting is a great way to detoxify your body. People spend a lot of money on vitamins, food supplements, and detoxifying cures just to get rid of the "hazardous waste" inside. Fasting works, guaranteed.

A fasting day may be followed by either another fasting day or a regular eating day. It's up to you to see how many fasting days you can commit to yourself. It can be as little as just one day a week or as many as seven days a week. The higher the level of commitment, the faster the results.

RESET YOUR WEIGHT THERMOSTAT

Did you ever go on a diet and successfully manage to lose some weight, but a few months later the pounds came back and you ended up weighing the same or even more than before? Why did that happen? Contrary to the widely-held belief, long-term weight loss is not just about counting calories. Your body desperately defends your preset weight. It looks like there is an invisible mechanism that keeps our body weight the same in the long run, just like the thermostat regulates the temperature of your house. If you ever experienced the yoyo dieting effect, you may be under the impression that our pre-programmed body weight is nearly impossible to change. It looks like the preset weight is "in your genes". Fortunately, this is not the case, at all. There is a solution, that works in the long run. Intermittent fasting is capable of resetting your body weight thermostat.

As mentioned earlier, my weight-loss program consists of a certain number of fasting days and regular eating days. It's totally up to you to decide how many fasting days you can commit yourself to. I recommend 24-hour fasting days followed by either

- a meal and another fasting day

or

-a regular eating day.

In the intense phase, when you start the program, try to do as many fasting days as you can. By doing that, you will enjoy two benefits at the same time: you will greatly speed up the weight-loss process and the fasting will reset your weight thermostat. We have already previously discussed that weight loss goes far beyond *calories consumed vs. calories expended*. Our weight is precisely regulated on a hormonal level, mainly by insulin. During fasting periods, insulin production pauses. As a result, the *insulin sensitivity* of your body's cells will greatly improve. If you repeat fasting days over and over again, you will gradually train your body to use insulin the right way: letting glucose inside the cells and using it as a fuel, instead of sending calories into your fat deposits. By fasting, you will slowly turn back the vicious cycle of *insulin resistance*, little by little, day by day.

PRACTICAL ADVICE

Fasting is the most efficient weapon in your battle against obesity. It works like the rocket engine of a space ship. Launching a spacecraft requires massive amounts of rocket fuel. However, space vehicles in orbit around the earth normally don't use any fuel. Occasionally, rocket engines are ignited for short periods of time to apply some minor corrections to the spacecraft's orbit, but most of the time, the rocket engines are shut down.

As you could figure out from this analogy, your ideal weight and health is like a space ship orbiting around our planet. Fasting is the rocket engine. Once you are in orbit, you don't need to fast anymore. There may be a few special occasions however, when you eat more than usual; you will have a fasting day thereafter, to get back "in orbit" again.

Let's see, how you can reach the ideal body weight, to get "in orbit". Intermittent fasting is your powerful rocket engine. To get started, I recommend the following protocol: fast every other day. On fasting days, refrain from food and caloric beverages for a period of 24 hours. Drink as much water as you want, and there is no limit on other, non-caloric beverage consumption either. At the end of your fast day, have a meal: select one dinner from the *"Weight-Loss Plans"* chapter. On eating days, choose one of the regular daily menus. Eat all the three meals within a period of 8 hours.

If you want faster results, increase the number of fasting days. For example, a 24-hour fasting is followed by a meal, then by another 24-hour fasting and finally you have an eating day. Repeat these patterns until you reach your target weight. Depending on your motivations, you can apply as many fasting days as you want. For example, I followed an even more rigorous protocol. I had eighty fasting days in a row: 24-hour fasting periods each followed by a meal. During that time, I achieved a nearly linear weight loss of more than half a pound a day: 42 pounds in 80 days (total weight loss of 55 pounds). Now, I weigh the same as I was back in high school. I don't even need to fast on a regular basis and just keeping the same weight without suffering.

FASTING IS NOT AS HARD AS IT SEEMS

Right before your regular dinner, you may feel terribly hungry. If you have never tried fasting before, you may assume that your hunger just gets worse and worse over time. This is absolutely wrong. The first pleasant surprise you will experience while fasting is that after a while hunger just disappears. Depending on the individual, it takes about half a day, and then no more hunger. The second surprise is that you are not much weaker than on a regular day. Some people even feel more energetic on fasting days. Once your glucose and glycogen supplies are depleted, your body gradually switches into fat burning. You can continue your regular daily job and even do physical exercise while you are fasting.

I'd like to emphasize that fasting and *calorie-restriction diets* are two totally different things. For example, if you just cut your caloric intake into half, you will be constantly hungry. You may slow down a lot and you will be very sluggish all day long. This happens because of the lower caloric intake; your body switches into an energy-saving mode. However, fasting is totally different.

Fasting has another positive health effect as well. Even after a one-day-fast, you will re-evaluate your way of thinking about food. In case if you were a picky eater before, you will appreciate ANY food. Another bonus is that fasting detoxifies your body. There is no need for any additional cures.

You may have heard from some diet "experts" about the long-term health effects of extended starvation periods. First of all, intermittent fasting is totally different from starvation. While you are doing intermittent fasting, you still have least one meal a day. Second, the body of overweight people stores large amounts of energy in the form of fat, that is enough to keep them alive for months. Even lean individuals have so much body fat, that – if all their energy deposits are mobilized – can keep them alive without food for a period of one month or two. You definitely won't starve to death in 24 hours. According to the *Guinness Book of World Records*, the longest recorded fast lasted for 382 days.

Experts say it takes three weeks to form a habit. Based on my own personal experience, it will happen much sooner. Even though in the beginning, fasting may seem a little bit challenging, after a couple of days, your body will quickly adapt to it. You will be surprised that fasting is not that hard at all. Fasting is a proven method that has been applied for thousands of years.

IF YOU ARE DIABETIC

However, if you are a diabetic, you need to be extra careful. Fasting is an extremely powerful tool to improve your insulin sensitivity.

Consult with your doctor in order to adjust your blood glucose-lowering medication. If your doctor opposes fasting, you may consider asking for a second opinion from a physician who is familiar with intermittent fasting. As mentioned earlier, a hundred years ago, Joslin successfully treated over 1,300 diabetic patients by applying dietary measures only. Otherwise, if you are not diabetic, fasting is absolutely safe for you.

46

THE RIGHT FOOD

WE WERE GIVEN BAD ADVICE

In 1977, the *Nutrition Committee of the United States Senate* formulated a paper entitled *Dietary Goals for the United States*. For the first time in U.S. history, the government told the citizens that they could improve their health by reducing their fat intake and increasing carbohydrate consumption in their diets. Americans did exactly what they were told to do: people cut back on fat and increased carbohydrate consumption. The 150-year-old wisdom of the fattening effect of carbohydrates got suddenly forgotten; all kinds of foods were called healthy, as long as they were low on fat. The 1991 pamphlet of the *American Heart Association* called the following foods healthy: white bread, hard candy, gum drops, sugar, syrup, honey, jam, jelly, marmalade, fruit punches and carbonated soft drinks. Even up to 12 ounces (0.36 liters) of beer (!) was on the list of the recommended healthy foods. A perfect recipe for disaster. No wonder that the introduction of the new dietary guidelines coincided with the beginning of the largest obesity epidemic in human history.

Readers may ask the question, how could such things happen? Why were we totally misinformed about carbohydrates for half a century? Didn't scientists warn us that refined carbohydrates cause obesity? Yes, they did. Actually, we have been continuously warned by scientists and doctors for the last 200 years. For example, the first one was *Brillat-Savarin* in the early 19th century; *Dr. Passmore* in 1963 or *Dr. Atkins* in 1972. However, since the 1970s, the *low-fat diet* became a political issue. The *low-fat – low-carb* debate was ended and won by politicians, not by scientists. Despite the lack of scientific evidence, heart disease was blamed on fat consumption and we were told to eat fat free, high-carbohydrate foods. The results are well known today.

Let's see why science and the whole healthcare system is corrupt to the core. The main reason is that scientific research is ultimately sponsored by the pharmaceutical and food industries. Here is a concrete example. Medical journals play a crucial role in the professional development of doctors, dieticians and the whole scientific research community. What is published in the leading medical journals has a great impact on the medical advice your physician will give you. Editors of these journals receive regular payments from the pharmaceutical industry.[64, 65] In return, those articles that prove the usefulness of a certain new drug are published, while those writings that don't favor the sponsors will be rejected.

Today's dietary guidelines are based on the 1992 publication of the *United States Department of Agriculture* (USDA), which is known as the *Food Pyramid*. Although the recommendations have been updated over the years, the *Food Pyramid* itself suffers from the same deficiency disease since its very inception: it's guidelines completely lack scientific evidence. The recommendations are based purely on politics, rather than on evidence-based science. The reason why the *Food Pyramid* is structured the way it is, is because politicians wanted to keep every segment of the food industry (a 5-trillion-dollar mega business) happy. It includes such powerful groups as the sugar lobby, the meat lobby, the dairy lobby, the cereal lobby, and so on. Figure 46.1 shows the *Food Pyramid*. If we take a quick look at the picture, those little triangle symbols represent added sugar. They are present in 4 of the 6 food groups. The USDA obviously encourages us to consume foods with added sugar (the impact of the mighty sugar lobby).

Cereals make up the first level of the pyramid. The authors recommend 6 to 11 servings of bread, cereal, rice and pasta, including those foods with added sugar. Unfortunately, the *Food Pyramid* does not distinguish between whole grain and highly processed cereal products. Whether grains are healthy or harmful greatly depends on the method of processing. You should eat whole grain cereals only. We need to completely avoid white flour, polished rice, and other

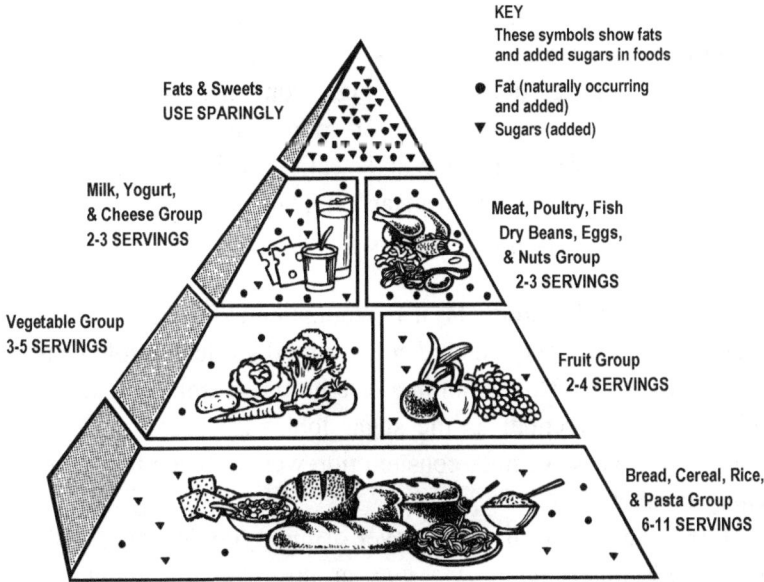

Figure 46.1. USDA Food Pyramid

highly processed grains that have had their bran and germ removed. These products have had the vast majority of the dietary fiber, protein and vitamin content extracted, and mills sell them separately as food supplements. Without these valuable nutrients, there is nothing left but starch. Without fiber's protective effects, the starch content of highly processed cereals is absorbed rapidly from the digestive tract and triggers an intense blood glucose and insulin response, which explains the fattening effect of refined carbohydrates.

Let's examine the *fruit group* on the next level. We were told to eat 2 to 4 servings a day. That's a lot of fruits. How do we know at all that fruits are really good for us? I think the main reason is that we were taught since the first year of kindergarten that fruits are healthy. Everybody looks at fruits as the symbol of healthy food choices and nobody is really questioning this dogma. Let's apply some critical thinking. Why are fruits very popular? Because they are so SWEET. The most popular ones include SWEET grapes, SWEET pineapples,

SWEET bananas and so on. Customers demand super-sweet tasting fruits. Those ones with less intense sweetness simply wouldn't sell, so they are not available in stores. Fruits are definitely not as bad as cakes or ice cream, but the high sugar content outweighs the health benefits of the nutritional value of antioxidants, minerals, vitamins and fiber. My recommendation is eating fruits only occasionally. Instead of fruits consume vegetables. They contain all the valuable nutrients with a negligible sugar content. Eat as many vegetables as you want.

Milk and dairy products: it is recommended to have 2 or 3 servings a day. I even encountered another food guide that told us to have 4 portions a day. This is nothing else but pure propaganda. The milk lobby is as influential as the sugar lobby is. The negative consequences of excessive milk consumption were detailed in the *Milk and Dairy* chapter.

Beside dairy, on the same level of the pyramid you can find the *meat, fish, beans, eggs and nuts* group. The only common thing among these foods is their high protein content. Otherwise, each one has a totally different effect on your health. We should distinguish between those foods; treating them together as a group is not a good idea.

Fats and sweets are on the top of the pyramid. The authors warn us to use them sparingly. We already discussed the topic in the *Dietary Fat* and *Beware of Sugar* chapters.

WHAT FOODS ARE HEALTHY?

Forget the Food Pyramid. The whole idea is based on pure politics rather than on scientific facts. The reason why the Food Pyramid is structured this way is that politicians wanted to keep every segment of the food industry happy, such as the sugar lobby, the meat lobby, the dairy lobby, the cereal lobby and so on. In addition to the food industry's dominance, the whole concept is based on an unproven theory: the *diet-heart hypothesis* that lacks scientific evidence.

In *Part IV* of this book, *Chapters 22 to 39* give you a detailed guide on nutrients; how to read food labels, which foods are good for you, and which ones should be avoided. If you haven't read these food guide chapters yet, it is a good idea to look up each nutrient group to get a better understanding of how food directly impacts our health. While healthy food is your best medicine, artificial food is like a poison for you.

CARBOHYDRATE FOODS

Official dietary guidelines encourage us to increase our carbohydrate consumption. In contrast, the Atkins diet and similar low-carb programs tell us to completely eliminate carbohydrates from our diet. Both approaches are equally wrong: they drastically oversimplify the complexity of the carbohydrates' role. We definitely need to distinguish between naturally occurring and refined / concentrated carbohydrates. Foods containing added sugar and highly processed grains are harmful. Without the protective effect of dietary fiber, the ingestion of refined carbohydrates results in a sudden spike in blood glucose levels followed by an insulin rush. Insulin is the main regulator of fat storage in our body. Elevated insulin levels divert nutrients into the fat deposits.

Unfortunately, the vast majority of commercially available foods is based on refined carbohydrates. Junk foods typically contain massive amounts of white flour, processed grains, and sugar. Sugar is present virtually in every single food item, even in those ones you wouldn't even suspect, such as in meat products, dairy, or vinegar. Our preference for sweet food is programmed in our mind since early childhood. Remember, we are all sugar addicts. In the *Blue Zones of* the world, the healthiest and longest living people don't use added sugar and highly refined carbohydrates. Sweets are reserved for holidays and special occasions only. You should do the same thing. Try to eliminate every single food with added sugar from your everyday diet. Use brown rice and whole grain flour instead. In the *Recipes* chapter of this book you will find detailed instructions on how to make your own healthy food.

I'd like to point out that commercially available breads, and those ones made from coarsely-ground, whole-wheat flour without sugar and additives, are two totally different foods. I personally recommend that every day you eat up to 250 grams (8 oz.) of bread or other bakery products that are made naturally, without sugar and additives, from *coarsely ground cereals*. This applies even for those with a sedentary lifestyle. If you don't like bread that much, you don't necessary need to eat 250 grams a day. You can replace bread with brown rice, beans and vegetables.

Beware of excessively sweet fruits. Even the organic ones are really bad for you. Eat fresh fruits only. Dried fruits have a very high sugar content. For example, dried dates may contain up to 66% of sugar.

Completely avoid sugar-sweetened beverages and fruit juices. In order to make them marketable, they must contain 10 to 12 % of sugar, even those ones with the "no added sugar" sticker. Foods with a high sugar content are bad for you.

Although artificial sweeteners contain nearly zero calories, they are even worse than sugar itself. Many of them are considered carcinogenic (cancer-causing) . Non-caloric sweeteners, similarly to real sugars, trigger a remarkable insulin response and they have a scientifically-proven fattening effect.

DIETARY FAT

The infamous 1977 paper entitled *Dietary Goals for the United States* had more severe impact on our health than any other dietary guidelines ever published. We were given bad advice. As a result of the cholesterol hysteria sweeping through the world in the 1970s, a low-fat, high-carbohydrate dietary pattern was forced on the whole population. As we gradually adopted the new dietary guidelines, we just became heavier and heavier.

You don't need to worry too much about dietary fat consumption. In *The Cholesterol Hysteria* chapter, we discussed in detail that dietary fat and cholesterol intake, and blood cholesterol levels are virtually independent of each other. Cholesterol is often confused with the low density lipoproteins known as LDL. It is also referred to as the "bad cholesterol". Although, there is some moderate correlation between LDL levels and cardiovascular disease, the relationship is much weaker than previously thought. Cholesterol itself is absolutely harmless, it plays many important functions and is present in every single cell of our body. Literally, there is no life without cholesterol. Every single day our body synthesizes approximately 700 milligrams of cholesterol. The more cholesterol you eat the less cholesterol your body has to produce. On the other hand, if you are on a low cholesterol diet, your body has to make more cholesterol than you would normally.

As a piece of practical advice, simply avoid extremes in fat consumption. A low-fat diet has no health benefits over a regular diet. Although the scientific evidence proving the *diet-heart hypothesis* is scant, there is still a very weak correlation between high saturated fat consumption and various diseases. Avoid foods with an excessively high fat content.

It doesn't make much difference if you eat lean or regular meat. However, don't use animal fat for cooking. Many researchers claim that it's palmitic acid content slightly increases LDL cholesterol. The results of different studies on animal fat consumption are controversial. Whether it is harmful or not, you cannot benefit from animal fats.

Omega-3 fatty acids have a remarkable cardioprotective and anti-inflammatory potential. In order to preserve your health, you should add omega-3 oils to your everyday diet. They easily break down if heated, therefore, use omega-3 oils to cold dishes and salads only, that don't require heating up the oil. The best sources of omega-3 oils include chia seeds, flax seeds and marine fish.

For general cooking purposes, I recommend extra virgin olive oil. Olive oil has been used for millennia and it is part of the traditional Mediterranian diet. The healthiest and longest living people in the *Blue Zones* cook with olive oil as well.

As a closing thought, another advice: don't use margarine or any other forms of industrially processed shortenings, especially hydrogenated fats. They just fall into the junk food category.

PROTEIN

Traditionally, meat was considered as a symbol of affluence. When a country's wealth grows, so does its meat consumption. As people eat more animal products, the prevalence rate of many civilization diseases increases parallelly with their meat intake. The United States is one of the largest red meat consumers in the world. Results of the latest research associated red meat consumption with an increased risk of serious disorders such as metabolic syndrome[103], cardiovascular disease, cancer[104] and diabetes[105]. Red meat products contain larger quantities of *heme* iron, which under certain circumstances, plays an important role in the formation of *free radicals* causing oxidative stress. This condition leads to a continuous low-grade inflammation in the body, which is associated with a whole range of diseases. Processed meat turned out to be even more harmful than red meat. During processing, meat is exposed to various chemicals such as nitrates, nitrites, phosphates and smoke.

Do you remember, what is common in the dietary habits of the longest-living-people of Sardinia, Icaria, Okinawa and Costa Rica? They have a predominantly plant-based diet and eat meat only occasionally. I am not trying to convince you to become a vegetarian. However, if meat is your staple food, you are in the high-risk group for developing a whole range of civilization diseases. The average meat consumption in Western countries is estimated between 200 and 250 pounds per person annually. To have that much meat, we need to eat the third of a cow, or 62 chickens. That's a lot of meat. If you are one of those "meatatarians", you may need to consider limiting your weekly meat intake to a maximum of 1 to 1.5 pounds. This amount can be served in small daily portions or 2 - 3 larger meals a week. Choose chicken or fish over red meat. The scientific explanations can be found in the *Animal Proteins* chapter of this book.

Although mother's milk is indispensable for babies since it contains all the necessary nutrients and immunoglobulins, adults and older children don't need milk at all. Health authorities however, keep on bombarding us with their message to have 2 or 3 glasses of milk every single day. I have to say that those vicious milk campaigns are nothing else but the propaganda of the influential milk lobby. The health benefits of regular milk consumption are based on anecdotal evidence only; they completely lack scientific proof. I'll go even further. Those countries with the highest per-capita milk consumption have the highest prevalence rates of a whole range of modern-day diseases, such as osteoporosis, cancer, cardiovascular disease, diabetes and others. In the *Milk and Dairy* chapter I gave detailed scientific explanation. If you are not a milk drinker, don't become one of them. If you can't live without milk and dairy, limit your intake to 1 or 2 servings a week.

Thanks to the worldwide epidemic of cholesterol hysteria, egg consumption in the United States has been declining since the 1970s. We shouldn't worry too much about dietary cholesterol however, because it has just a minimal effect on LDL cholesterol levels. Although eggs by themselves are high in cholesterol, egg consumption doesn't significantly affect blood cholesterol levels. You can safely eat eggs; prepare them the way you like.

Plant proteins are a healthy alternative for meat. All the necessary amino acids that are present in meat can be supplied from plant food as well. There are 20 naturally occurring amino acids, and 10 of them are called essential, which means the body can not synthesize them. There are only four *limiting amino acids* that have a particular importance in the protein synthesis in our body: *lysine, methionine, threonine* and *tryptophan*. With regular consumption of whole grains and legumes all of our essential amino acid requirements are met. Rich plant sources of protein include beans, peas, chickpeas, peanuts, walnuts, almonds, mung beans, chia seeds and lentils. Eat them as often as you can.

DIETARY FIBERS

To the indispensable role of dietary fibers, I dedicated a whole chapter, entitled *Man's Best Friend*. Dietary fibers have numerous health benefits, including reducing the risk of developing some cancers, hyperlipidemia, hypertension, coronary heart disease and type-2 diabetes. Dietary fibers greatly slow down the absorption rate of carbohydrates and reduce the post-meal insulin response. As a result of lower insulin levels, fewer calories will be deposited in fat cells.

Although I am not an advocate of a raw food diet, I recommend that you prepare your food with a minimal degree of processing. Those fruits and vegetables that are edible raw or semi-raw, should be consumed that way. Leafy vegetables are an excellent source of fibers. Don't cook them or put them into a blender to turn them into a liquid. Cooking increases the digestibility and glycemic index of vegetables and diminishes dietary fiber's protective effects.

SUMMARY

Everybody knows the old saying: "You are what you eat". There is a lot of truth in this proverb. While healthy food is your medicine, bad food acts like a poison. The choice is entirely in your hands. Eating the right food is the second building block of a successful and permanent weight-loss program.

The objective of this chapter was to give you a brief overview on how to choose wisely from the main nutrient groups. *Part IV* of the book gives you a more detailed description on the health effects of various food items, which ones are good for your health, and which ones should be avoided.

47

PHYSICAL ACTIVITY

THE CALORIES IN, CALORIES OUT MYTH

The official formula for weight loss sounds like this: eat less, exercise more. The vast majority of mainstream scientists believe that obesity is just a result of a caloric imbalance between calories consumed and calories expended. In order to lose a certain amount of weight, the only thing you need to do is either to decrease your caloric intake or increase your physical activity level. The missing calories in your energy balance will be automatically taken away from your fat deposits. WRONG! Most of us have already tried cutting back on meals or doing some form of exercising once in a while. Honestly, did it work? If calorie counting was an efficient weight-loss method in real life, you probably wouldn't be reading this book.

In contrast, many exercise deniers are questioning the usefulness of physical activities as a weight-loss tool at all. They argue that you can't simply lose weight by exercising, because being involved in physical activities will increase your appetite. At the end of the day instead of burning fat, you will even have a positive energy balance. Both approaches are equally wrong. Let's see why.

From the *calories in-calories out* view point, being involved in strenuous physical exercise is an extremely inefficient solution for weight loss. For example, a small, 25-gram chocolate chip cookie contains 122 kcal of energy. To burn these excess calories you have to sweat in the gym for 15 minutes or walk for half an hour. It is definitely not worth it. Exercise deniers claim that vigorous physical exercise or outdoor activities may ultimately lead to an increased appetite. At the end of the day, instead of losing you will end up even gaining some weight. I think this statement is not necessarily true.

Whether certain sport activities increase appetite or not, greatly depends on the individual and the type of physical exercise.

In addition to the problem of increased appetite, there is another adverse effect of exercising as well. If you do your exercise in the morning, your metabolic rate will noticeably slow down; you will be a little bit sluggish for the rest of the day and will spend less energy on other activities. As a result, your net energy balance will be zero. In other words, according to the calories in-calories out model, you may not lose weight at all.

WHY DO WE NEED TO EXERCISE?

From the conventional *calories in-calories out* viewpoint, physical exercise has zero, or just a minimal weight-loss effect. As we concluded, if we look at the number of expended calories only, exercising is definitely not worth it. However, the *calories in-calories out* model turned out to be incorrect. For a detailed explanation, see *The Importance of Exercising* chapter. Let's focus on the most important question: Is exercising necessary at all? I have really bad news for you: the answer is definitely yes. Let's see why.

Both obesity and type-2 diabetes have the same underlying cause: insulin resistance. Physical exercise significantly improves the body's insulin sensitivity. Continuous muscle contractions facilitate glucose uptake by the cells. As a result of improved insulin sensitivity, the pancreas has to secrete lower amounts of the hormone. Having lower insulin levels means we gain less weight.

Direct calorie burning is just a less important, secondary effect. Regular physical exercise helps you break down fat tissue and build lean muscle mass. Muscle tissue has a higher metabolic rate than fat tissue. Even if your body weight doesn't change much, you still burn more energy.

A physically active lifestyle greatly reduces the risk factors for a series of life-threatening diseases such as coronary heart disease, stroke, thrombosis, type-2 diabetes and cancer. Regular physical exercise also plays an important role in the prevention of arthritis, osteoporosis, dementia and depression.

HOW MUCH EXERCISE DO I NEED?

The world's healthiest people live a physically active life. In order to stay in good shape, *Blue Zones* people don't need to go to the gym, however. They do long-lasting, low intensity physical work instead, such as gardening and household chores, which keep them busy all the day. If you work as a brickmason, carpenter or roofer, you probably don't need any extra physical exercise. However, for those of us who are less physically active, especially those who have a sedentary lifestyle, regular exercising plays an important role in preserving our health.

As discussed earlier, the *direct* fat-burning effects of exercising are negligible. However, being involved in regular physical activities significantly increases the body's insulin sensitivity, making physical exercise indispensable for your health. You don't need to sweat in the gym for long hours. Of course, you can still do it if you want to, but it's not necessary. If you have a sedentary lifestyle, half an hour of a medium-intensity workout every day will do the job for you. You can do any sport you like that keeps your heart rate high enough throughout the whole workout session. The emphasis is on the continuously elevated heart rate. For example, ball games don't count if you are a goalkeeper or your activity level drops down during the session. Swimming is absolutely the very best choice. It improves your cardiovascular health; it is an all-over body workout, as nearly all of your muscles are used during swimming. It improves muscle tone and maintains bone health. Swimming is also an excellent stress reliever. Being obese or overweight may hinder some people participating in physical exercise. Fortunately, that's not the case with swimming. Besides swimming, there are many other good choices as well: jogging, walking briskly, biking, zumba, dancing, stair climbing or treadmill exercise. Any type of workout is good for you, as long as it keeps your heart rate continuously high.

HOW TO GET STARTED

If you suffer from cardiovascular disease or have other serious medical conditions, you need to consult with your doctor first. If you are healthy, you can go ahead with your training program. The first step is to make the decision to begin. If you already did that, you're on your way to a healthier life. Next, set your ultimate goal: half an hour of medium-intensity exercise at least 5 or 6 times a week. If you can exercise every day, even better. Skeptics may be wondering: Is it good enough to work out only once or twice a week? Let me ask you a question: do you want to live a healthy life one or two days a week, or every single day? We should keep in mind, that besides an unhealthy diet, virtually every single modern-day civilization disease is closely related to a sedentary lifestyle.

You need to incorporate regular physical exercise into your every-day life. If you have a sedentary lifestyle, in the beginning you may find it a little bit challenging. However, if you exercise diligently, after a short period of time you will get used to it. Experts say, it takes three weeks to form a habit. Once it becomes a part of your life, you will even miss every single occasion if you weren't able to exercise for some reason. You just need to make a decision to commit half an hour of your time each day to be healthy in the long run.

If you haven't regularly exercised before, take the advice to "start low and go slow." Many beginners make the mistake of starting out too aggressively. They may end up tired or injured and are most like-ly to quit. Your ultimate goal is to develop some new habits that you can stick with for a lifetime. If you are an absolute beginner, start with 10-15 minutes of workout. Gradually increase the intensity and the length of each session every week. Any little increment in your physical activity level will significantly improve your overall health. It may take a couple of months until you gain enough strength to complete those half an hour medium-intensity sessions.

As a piece of practical advice, try to do your workouts in the late afternoon or evening hours. If evening exercising doesn't interfere with your sleep, do it as late as possible. If you exercise early morn-ing, you may feel tired for the rest of the day. It may slow down your metabolic rate and as a result you will spend less energy throughout the rest of the day.

48

OTHER WEIGHT-LOSS FACTORS

REDUCE YOUR STRESS LEVEL

In the previous chapters, we saw the three most important aspects of a successful weight-loss program: *when to eat*, *what to eat* and the role of *physical exercise*. Let's see what other factors influence whether you lose or gain weight.

Lifestyle diseases are both directly and indirectly linked to our stressful, modern-day life. Long-term stress exposure not only makes you sick but also causes weight gain. The stress hormone *cortisol* is one of the major regulators of our fat metabolism. Elevated cortisol levels cause the formation of fat deposits, especially in the abdominal area. Here is some practical advice. Most importantly, you need to slow down. Avoid stressful situations if possible. Make sure you get an adequate amount of sleep. Exercise regularly. Working out is the best stress relief. You can benefit from regular physical exercise in multiple ways. First, participating in physical activities significantly increases your insulin sensitivity. Second, during exercise sessions you also burn some calories. Third, you improve your overall health. Fourth, if you exercise regularly, you will sleep better. Fifth, as already mentioned, working out helps you to get rid of your everyday stress.

It is very hard to lose weight without getting a healthy amount of sleep. Sleep deprivation increases your cortisol levels. Cortisol is a long-term stress hormone. As an adaptive response to continuous stress exposure, the human body builds up fat deposits typically in the abdominal regions. This is the type of obesity that everybody wants to avoid. Make sure you get at least 7 or 8 hours of sleep.

It is a scientifically proven fact, that keeping a pet has numerous health benefits. Pet owners have a significantly reduced risk for cardiovascular disease, depression, and hypertension. Looking after other living things is a great way of relieving your everyday stress. If you have a backyard, try gardening. Taking care of your plants not only reduces your stress level, but also engages you in some physical exercise and you can also grow some organic vegetables for free.

Spend as much time as you can on outdoor activities. Go fishing, hiking, bird watching or whatever activities you like. In addition to these health benefits, as little as 10-15 minutes of exposure to sunlight covers your entire daily vitamin D requirements.

CHECK YOUR WEIGHT REGULARLY

Researchers found that individuals weighing themselves every day, lose more weight than those who don't check their weight very often. Checking your weight daily may be an extremely strong motivating factor for you, as it gives you regular feedback on the effectiveness of your weight-loss plan.

First, you need to invest into a reliable scale. The old fashioned *medical beam scales* are the most accurate ones, however they are quite expensive. If you don't want to spend that much, digital scales with an accuracy of 0.5 pounds or 0.2 kg will be the right ones for you. Weighing yourself first thing in the morning is the best practice. Keep a record of your weight loss. Don't be discouraged if you experience some "plateaus" in your weight loss. There are many possible reasons why your weight did not go down as expected. As a result of regular, strenuous exercising, your weight may remain constant while you are still burning fat and building up muscle mass. If you drink lots of fluids or eat salty foods, your body weight will temporarily increase as a consequence of water retention. This is not permanent, however. Women also may experience some temporary weight gain during their period.

49

WEIGHT-LOSS PLANS

WEIGHT-LOSS AND WEIGHT-MAINTENANCE DAYS

As discussed in *The Eating Window* chapter, your regimen consists of *fasting days* (weight-loss days) and regular *eating days* (weight-maintenance days). On fasting days no food is allowed, but there is no limit on non-caloric fluid intake. The typical length of a fasting period is 24 hours. A fasting day may be followed by either

-a meal and another fasting day

or

-a regular eating day.

My weight-loss program is very flexible: it is built up in a modular system. It's up to you to see how many fasting days you can commit to. It can be as little as just one day a week or as many as seven days a week. The higher the level of commitment, the faster the results. In the beginning, when you start the program, you will have a relatively higher number of weight-loss days. Later, when you are at your target weight, your regimen typically contains *weight maintenance days* only. The whole method is self-sustaining. You can even go through several months without having one single fasting day. On special occasions however, when you have a dinner with friends and family, you probably eat more than usual. These days are typically followed by a *weight-loss day*.

On *weight maintenance days* you eat three meals; the time period between the first and the last meal of the day should not be longer than 8-10 hours.

To those, who are just getting started, I recommend an alternating-style eating pattern: each *weight-loss day* is followed by a *weight maintenance day*. Of course, you can increase the number of your *weight-loss days,* if you want faster results. You will find sample weight-loss plans later in this chapter.

FOODS TO BE AVOIDED

Refined carbohydrates are the number one cause of today's world-wide obesity epidemic. Completely avoid every single food item that contains added sugar, white flour and white rice. Avoid corn and potatoes. Keep away from excessively sweet fruits, dried fruits, sugar-sweetened beverages, ketchup, fruit juices and beer. Don't consume any artificial sweeteners. Read the ingredient list on food labels carefully: they may be a little bit tricky in some countries. Please refer to the *How to Read Food Labels* chapter.

LIMIT THE CONSUMPTION OF THESE FOOD ITEMS

In the *Animal Proteins* chapter we discussed in detail that the intake of excessive amounts of animal proteins is associated with a whole range of diseases. Although strictly from the viewpoint of weight-loss purposes, proteins are definitely better than carbohydrates, the overconsumption of animal proteins has proven negative health effects over time.

Try to limit your weekly meat intake to a maximum of 1 to 1.5 pounds. This amount can be served in small daily portions or 2 or 3 larger meals a week. Choose chicken or fish over red meat. Limit your daily egg consumption to 3 eggs; prepare them the way you like. If you don't consume milk and dairy at all, that is fine. If you can't live without milk and dairy, limit the intake to 1 or 2 servings a week. Don't eat sweet fruits at all. Those varieties with a moderate sugar content are recommended for up to two or three servings a week. Choose vegetables instead. They contain all the valuable nutri-ents that fruits have with a much lower sugar content. There is one exception: I recommend one apple a day. Choose the less sweet vari-eties, such as *Mcintosh.*

YOUR HEALTHY FOOD CHOICES

The healthiest and longest living people in the world have a predominantly plant-based diet. Although they are not vegetarians, they consume significantly less meat than Westerners do. You should adopt a similar eating pattern. For baking and cooking use coarse, whole-grain flour only. Select rice varieties with a low glycemic index. Long-grain brown rice is the healthiest choice, for example brown basmati rice.

With regular consumption of whole grains and legumes, all our protein requirements are met. Rich plant sources of protein include beans, peas, chickpeas, peanuts, walnuts, almonds, mung beans, chia and lentils.

Eat all sorts of vegetables, as many as you can. Adding cabbage to your meal promotes the feeling of fullness. Kale is one of the world's healthiest foods. Consider kale as the secret weapon in your battle against obesity. Add at least 3 or 4 leaves of kale to your diet every single day. Always eat it raw, don't turn it into a liquid in a blender. Prepare it the way you like.

You don't need to reduce your total fat intake. However, make sure to eat the healthy ones. For cooking, always use extra-virgin olive oil. You also need to pay attention to getting enough *omega-3 fatty acids*. They can be found in fatty marine fish, chia seeds, and flax seed oil.

Use any spices you like, as much as you want. Their health benefits are inexhaustible. A salt-free diet is not good for your health. You can add salt to every food you like, but use it moderately. Vinegar helps you lose weight. Consume at least 3 to 5 tablespoons of vinegar every day. Always read labels. Buy only those vinegars that contain no sugar.

Make sure you are always well-hydrated. Drink as much water as you like. Coffee and tea consumption is fine, but don't add any sugar, artificial sweeteners or milk.

Dietary iodine plays an important role in maintaining adequate thyroid gland functions. Seaweed is a very rich, natural source of iodine and many other valuable nutrients including vitamin B_{12}. For example, our daily iodine requirement can be satisfied by 4 grams of dried *nori*. Instead of using iodized salt, which also contains chemical additives, adding seaweed to our diet is a healthy alternative.

For more information visit the author's website. Scan the code on the right with your device.

THREE MEALS A DAY PLANS

Similarly to traditional eating patterns, you'll have three meals a day. However, the main difference is that instead of starting with a plentiful breakfast early in the morning, you are encouraged to eat your breakfast as late as you can and the last meal of the day as early as possible. The main goal is to narrow down the eating window, the timeframe between the first and the last meals of the day, to 8-10 hours. Do not snack between meals. Remember, while you are fasting, instead of building new fat deposits, your body burns calories from it's own energy reserves.

Table 49.1 shows a week's weight maintenance regimen. For more details on each food please visit the *Recipes* chapter. The menu you can find in this weekly plan is not mandatory, it was meant to give you just some rough ideas. You can replace any of those meals with your own choices. Before adding new items to your menu, review the earlier chapters carefully to see which foods are good for you and which ones are harmful. You can find lots of useful information on various food items throughout chapters 23 to 39. Don't forget, healthy food is even more powerful than any kind of medicine.

The regimen does not specify serving sizes. You may ask the question: How much food should I eat? The answer greatly depends on the individual. I recommend that you follow the 80 percent rule. The Okinawans in Japan, who belong to the healthiest and longest living people in the world call it *hara hachi bu*, which means eat until you are 80 percent full. To avoid temptations, serve yourself the exact amount of food you will eat; don't go for a second serving.

Day	Breakfast	Lunch	Dinner
1	Scrambled eggs Bread Vegetables Tea	Smoked salmon Bread Olives Feta cheese	Lentil soup Grilled chicken Brown rice Mixed salad
2	Omelet with mushrooms Bread Tea	Chickpea salad Boiled eggs Bread	Green pea soup Fried salmon Brown rice Mixed salad
3	Muesli with bananas and pears	Fried eggs Bread Vegetables Tea	Chicken soup Fried chicken Brown rice Mixed salad
4	Omelet with pepper and tomatoes Bread, tea	Fried mushrooms Green beans	Pumpkin soup Fried trout Brown rice Mixed salad
5	Fried eggs Bread Vegetables Tea	Canned sardines Bread Tomato salad Chives	Bean soup Indian chicken Brown rice Mixed salad
6	Muesli with mixed berries	Greek salad Boiled eggs Bread Tea	Split pea soup Fried tilapia Brown rice Mixed salad
7	Omelet with vegetables Bread Tea	Homemade pizza with toppings of your choice	Mushroom soup Fried cod Brown rice Mixed salad

Table 49.1. Sample weekly weight maintenance plan

Day	Breakfast	Lunch	Dinner
1	Scrambled eggs Bread Vegetables Tea	Smoked salmon Bread Olives Feta cheese	Lentil soup Grilled chicken Brown rice Mixed salad
2	Fast day Fluid intake only	Fast day Fluid intake only	Green pea soup Fried salmon Brown rice Mixed salad
3	Omelet with pepper and tomatoes Bread, tea	Fried mushrooms Green beans	Chicken soup Fried chicken Brown rice Mixed salad
4	Fast day Fluid intake only	Fast day Fluid intake only	Pumpkin soup Fried trout Brown rice Mixed salad
5	Fried eggs Bread Vegetables Tea	Canned sardines Bread Tomato salad Chives	Bean soup Indian chicken Brown rice Mixed salad
6	Fast day Fluid intake only	Fast day Fluid intake only	Split pea soup Fried tilapia Brown rice Mixed salad
7	Omelet with vegetables Bread Tea	Homemade pizza with toppings of your choice	Mushroom soup Fried cod Brown rice Mixed salad

Table 49.2. Sample 1-1 weight-loss plan

Day	Breakfast	Lunch	Dinner
1	Scrambled eggs Bread Vegetables Tea	Smoked salmon Bread Olives Feta cheese	Lentil soup Grilled chicken Brown rice Mixed salad
2	Fast day Fluid intake only	Fast day Fluid intake only	Green pea soup Fried salmon Brown rice Mixed salad
3	Fast day Fluid intake only	Fast day Fluid intake only	Chicken soup Fried chicken Brown rice Mixed salad
4	Omelet with pepper and tomatoes Bread, tea	Fried mushrooms Green beans	Pumpkin soup Fried trout Brown rice Mixed salad
5	Fast day Fluid intake only	Fast day Fluid intake only	Bean soup Indian chicken Brown rice Mixed salad
6	Fast day Fluid intake only	Fast day Fluid intake only	Split pea soup Fried tilapia Brown rice Mixed salad
7	Omelet with vegetables Bread Tea	Homemade pizza with toppings of your choice	Mushroom soup Fried cod Brown rice Mixed salad

Table 49.3. Sample 1-2 weight-loss plan

Table 49.2 shows a week's *weight-loss plan*. The only difference between this plan and the *weight-maintenance plan* from the previous table is that breakfast and lunch are omitted every other day. On fasting days, you don't eat for 24 hours, then you have dinner and the following day is a regular eating day (1-1 plan). You can have your dinner on fasting days any time of the day, it doesn't have to be in the evening, as long as you have been fasting for at least 24 hours.

For quicker results, you can increase the number of weekly fast days. Table 49.3 shows a 1-2 regimen (one eating day – two fasting days). As mentioned before, the plan is built up in a modular system. It's up to you to see how many fasting days you can commit to. It can be as little as just one day a week or as many as seven days a week. The higher the level of commitment, the faster the results. Regardless of what plan you follow, you will still have at least one meal every 24 hours, and you won't be starving. Here is my own testimony: I was on an 80-day *all fasting day protocol* and managed to lose 42 pounds during that period of time (55 pounds in total) .

NIGHT OWLS' SECRET WEAPON

There are individuals, who are not hungry in the morning at all but simply can not fall asleep with an empty stomach. I call them *night owls*. Being a night owl has a disadvantage: eating late at night leads to obesity. We discussed earlier that the same food has a significantly less fattening effect if consumed in the morning rather then late at night. Therefore, we should have the last meal of the day as early as possible. If such a late-night eating pattern sounds familiar to you, there is a good chance that you are a night owl as well. My first advice for night owls is that they should make some reasonable efforts to follow a regular eating pattern and avoid night-eating. That may work for some individuals, while others simply can not change their daily routine.

Mainstream nutrition science cannot really address this issue. Forcing night people to have a plentiful breakfast early in the morning when they aren't hungry at all is not a good idea. It will significantly extend the feeding period of the day, and as a result, they will never lose weight. I haven't mentioned yet, I am a typical night owl type myself. I have successfully used the following protocol since 2016.

In order to avoid the temptation of visiting the fridge after midnight, I created a solution for the problem of night-eating. On eating days, have your breakfast at noon or even at 1 PM. Skip lunch. Have your dinner at 8 PM. At 10 PM, eat 4 ounces of *whole-wheat scones* (see recipe section). Chew them very slowly and drink a big glass of ice cold water in between. By doing so, the fiber-rich, whole-wheat scone and the ice cold water, will give you an extended feeling of fullness. By the way, home-made, *whole-wheat scones* taste really good. Once you are done, have an apple that is not sweet. In addition to the benefits of the whole-grains, and the apple's soluble fiber content, you will also get the advantage of the *second meal phenomenon*: if a meal is followed by another meal within a few hours, the second meal has a diminished fattening effect. For detailed explanations see *What to Eat vs. When to Eat chapter.*

The weight-loss days for night owls are the same as in the early bird schedule: a 24-hour fasting followed by a meal.

50

HOW TO PREPARE YOUR FOOD

THE THIRTY-DAY RULE

Ancient civilizations accumulated and preserved the human wisdom of millennia. There is an old Greek saying that is attributed to *Hippocrates*, the father of medicine: "Let food be thy medicine and medicine be thy food". Unfortunately, this principle is not really applied today. We live in an unhealthy environment and eat unnatural, engineered foods, mass produced in factories. The vast majority of our modern-day civilization diseases could be prevented by simply adopting a healthy lifestyle. In the long run, food is the most important factor determining whether you will be sick or healthy. Unfortunately, today's profit-oriented food industry is not really concerned about your health. I just call this phenomenon the *30-day rule*. Big and powerful corporations are not really ashamed of selling you anything harmful if you won't die from their product within 30 days.

TAKE BACK CONTROL OF YOUR LIFE

You need to take back control of your life in order to be healthy. As the first step, completely eliminate *junk food* from your diet. The meaning of *junk food* is not limited to hot dogs, ice cream and sugary soft drinks. The vast majority of highly-processed foods that you can buy in junk food restaurants or grocery stores fall into the *engineered food* category, or garbage. These foods are not real ones: they are not cooked in a kitchen, but are manufactured in large factories. Their recipes have been continuously developed by the brilliant food scientists of the biggest international companies for decades. Engineered food products are neither healthy nor satisfying. The *Big Food*

Industry has one goal only: to increase their sales figures, even at the expense of your health.

Finding genuinely healthy foods in stores and restaurants is not an easy task. Only a few items will meet our criteria. Besides, healthy food may be very pricy, being well over your budget. Why don't you try making your own food instead? By doing that, you will have 100% control over the food you eat. You don't need to worry anymore about added sugar, trans fat, artificial sweeteners, cancer-causing chemicals, MSG, preservatives, or any other hidden ingredients. Instead of factory-made artificial food, you can make your own from natural ingredients like whole-wheat flour, brown rice, fresh vegetables, fruits, meat and fish. No worries if you are not a cooking expert. I'll explain everything step-by-step, from scratch. I will teach you the tricks to prepare your healthy and delicious food in no time. Just keep on reading this chapter and the next one with the recipes.

In addition to the health benefits and better taste of real, home made food, it will also cost you significantly less than eating out in junk food restaurants. If you do some quick math, you will see that eating the healthy way will actually cost you less than being on junk food.

THE CRIME OF REFINED CARBOHYDRATES

The whole, modern food industry is built on refined carbohydrates, predominantly on sugar and starch. In the chapter entitled *"Beware of Sugar"* I already discussed how sugar, similarly to alcohol, causes addiction. Junk food manufacturers are well aware of that fact. By taking the advantage of our sugar addiction, they put sugar in virtually ever food item. If you thoroughly go through your food labels, you will be shocked that even those foods where you wouldn't ever suspect it, contain sugar. For example, meat products, breads, or vinegars may contain a considerable amount of sugar, in order to make them more appealing to sugar addicts.

The adverse health effect of white flour has been known for 200 years. American preacher, *Sylvester Graham* launched America's first food protest movement. Graham pointed out that white flour coming from the new mills was unhealthy and began advocating for the consumption of locally-produced, whole-grain wheat flour.

Beside easy workability, there are two other good reasons why food manufacturers prefer highly-refined, white flour over the wholesome, whole-grain flour. First, the production cost of white flour is lower (it is produced on a larger scale; also the bran and germ portion of the kernels are sold by mills separately). The second problem is even bigger. Natural, coarsely-ground, whole-wheat flour makes very satisfying foods. You need to eat just half the amount of white flour products to have the same feeling of fullness. This is a very serious issue. Imagine if *Big Food* lost 50% of their sales! Food companies are well aware of that. Probably, that's why for the last century or two, we were trained from early childhood to prefer white flour and sugar-based food.

It's time to start your first food protest movement. As step 1, grab an extra large garbage bag. You probably will need even more than one. Go through your pantry, fridge, and freezer. Carefully read the labels of every single food item. Throw out everything that contains added sugar, white flour and white rice. Once you are done, you may find your pantry and fridge in a nearly empty state. If you haven't convinced your family members yet, to stay out of trouble, be careful not to put their food into the garbage for now. Do your best to persuade every single person in your household that living on an unhealthy diet has serious consequences for their health in the future. Put a health risk warning sticker on every single junk food item that didn't end up in the garbage for some reason. You can design your own stickers, or order from the author's website. See figure 50.1.

www.thepermanentweightloss.com

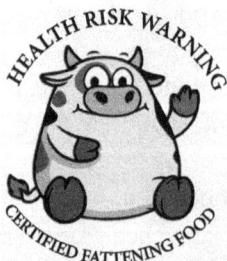

Figure 50.1. Health Risk Warning sticker. Tag every single remaining junk food item in your home in order to draw everybody's attention in your household to the fact that junk food is unhealthy and leads to obesity.

Once you get rid of the most harmful food stuff in your kitchen, it's time to go shopping. For wholesome food, you need wholesome ingredients.

WHOLESOME GRAINS

Rice varieties may look pretty similar to the non-experts. It is important to know however, that the glycemic index of a white rice may be twice as high as the glycemic index of a good variety. Always choose unpolished, long-grain brown rice. The best ones are *Basmati* and *Doongara* varieties. Basmati rice is available in many Asian food stores. If you can not find it, go with any other type of long-grain, brown rice.

Purchasing the right flour is a little bit more of a challenging task. Most commercially available flours are detrimental to your health. What's wrong with them? Everything. First, they are made from the wrong wheat varieties. Second, during the milling process all bran and germ are removed. Third, the kernels are ground into fine dust particles, turning flour into a high glycemic index food. Fourth, the flour is bleached with chemical additives. Fifth, bakeries mix further chemicals into the dough. Isn't that scary enough?

What does a wholesome bakery product look like? Exactly the same way as it did 200 years ago. The flour was made from ancient wheat varieties like *Einkorn* or *Emmer*. The flour was ground coarse and not turned into fine, dust-like particles. It has no additives. Bread should have four ingredients only: flour, water, yeast / leaven and salt. Because making such healthy bread is not really a profitable business, it is not commercially available in most parts of the world.

There are two solutions to how you can make your natural, wholesome bread. You can either use *Graham flour*, which is a coarse-ground, whole-wheat flour or make your own flour. If you decide to go with the second option, you need to buy a small milling machine first. To test your flour, you can also use an electric coffee grinder, but for larger quantities you need more professional equipment. Shop online for *"Wondermill"*. It is very fast and quite reliable, I have been using mine for years. To produce the right flour on *Wondermill*, turn the button into the position between *medium* and *coarse*. *Einkorn* and *Emmer* are two ancient wheat varieties especially rich in fiber, protein, minerals and vitamins. They are typically not available in health food stores, but some organic farms sell them online. *Spelt* is the third ancient wheat variety I recommend. If none of these three are available in your area, use *rye* or *barley*.

For more information on how to make your wholesome, all natural bread, visit the recipe section of the book. Although making your own bread may seem a little bit challenging, it is definitely worth it. In addition to its numerous health benefits, homemade natural bread has an exceptional taste. Once you try it, you will never want the supermarket bread again.

FRUITS AND VEGETABLES

Most importantly, don't buy fruits and vegetables in their processed form, for example pre-cooked vegetables, fruit juices, jams, dried fruits or ready meals. Prepare your food from raw fruits and vegetables instead. Those ones that are edible raw or semi-raw, should be eaten that way. Otherwise cook them with a minimal degree of processing. Although frozen fruits and vegetables are not the perfect solution, they are still acceptable if they were not processed before freezing. Always dispose of the juices that leak out, after the fruits and vegetables are thawed, because these liquids are relatively high in sugars.

MEAT AND FISH

Completely avoid highly-processed meats, fish and other animal products. During manufacturing, meat is exposed to harmful chemicals like nitrates, nitrites and phosphates. Prepare your meat and seafood the way you like, but always use fresh ingredients. There is one exception however: canned fish. Sardines are rich in omega-3 fatty acids. As a general rule, avoid every kind of canned fish, except for sardines in water. Drain the water after opening the can. Add one or two tablespoons of *flaxseed oil*, another excellent source of omega-3 fatty acids.

USE SPICES AS MUCH AS YOU LIKE

Spices in your food are just like colors for your eyes: they make life more enjoyable. Don't be shy; if you don't find the following recipes flavorful enough, feel free to add your own spices as much as you want. The health benefits of spices and herbs are inexhaustible

PRACTICAL ADVICE

Making your own healthy food is much easier than you think. If you are well-organized, it shouldn't take longer than a couple of hours a week. First of all, you don't need to cook every day. Make 5-10 portions every time you prepare something, and put the food in serving-sized containers into your freezer. Place into each box the exact amount of food you will eat for one meal. Half a day before you need it, take one container out of the freezer and let it sit at room temperature. Gently microwave it in a glass or porcelain bowl right before you eat. Never put any plastic containers or bags in microwave oven. Make sure you don't place more food into the containers than your serving size. This practice will prevent you from the temptation of overeating, since the rest of your food is in the freezer.

If you have ever experienced the taste and smell of freshly baked, homemade bread, you will never buy those cheap bread imitations from supermarkets that taste just like sawdust. I will tell you the secret of how you can enjoy the goodness of fresh bread any time you want, without making bread every single day. Fortunately, you can freeze your homemade bread without compromising its freshness and nutritional value. The fact of the matter is, that freezing even further improves the quality of your bread. Frozen bread has a lower glycemic index than fresh bread.[153] Cut your bread into serving-sized pieces and freeze them. When needed, just take a piece out of your freezer and let it sit at room temperature for 2-3 hours before mealtime. It will taste just like you've taken it out of the oven. Freezing is an excellent solution to preserve the freshness of other bakery products as well such as wheat scones or pizza.

As a closing thought, here is some practical advice on how to avoid overeating. Most importantly, always eat a fixed-size serving and don't go back for a second plate. If you store your food in one-serving-sized container in your freezer, and thaw only one box per meal, you won't have access to other food and can easily avoid the temptation of eating more than your regular portion. To determine portion sizes, eat until you are 80 percent full; the Japanese call it the *hara hachi bu* rule.

Eating some cabbage before your regular dinner gives you a satisfying feeling of fullness and as a result you will eat less food. You can have *sauerkraut*, a few leaves of raw cabbage or pan-fried cabbage. Kale is one of the world's healthiest foods, make it a cornerstone of your everyday diet. Eat as much kale as you can: chew on a few raw kale leaves before your dinner or make a kale salad.

The next chapter is a concise cookbook with a collection of recipes that don't require any special skills. Those foods are very easy to prepare, are nutritious, and taste good too.

51

RECIPES

TEA

Pick your favorite tea variety
Always use *loose leaf tea* instead of teabags
Pour hot water into a mug
Place tea leaves in a small strainer and put it into the mug for 2-3 minutes
Enjoy your tea with no sugar, sweetener or milk
Optionally you can add a slice of lemon, a piece of cinnamon or a few cardamom seeds

FRIED EGGS

Heat 1 tablespoon of olive oil in a pan over low-medium heat
Crack 3 eggs
Fry the eggs until they reach the desired hardness
Top with some salt and spices of your choice (such as ground pepper or paprika powder)

SCRAMBLED EGGS

Heat 2 tablespoons of olive oil in a pan over medium heat
Whisk 3 eggs and a pinch of salt together in a small bowl
Pour the egg mixture into the pan
As eggs begin to set, gently move spatula across the bottom to break the egg curds that begin to form in the pan
Cook until no visible liquid egg remains

SCRAMBLED EGGS WITH ONIONS

Dice a medium sized onion into small cubes
Whisk 3 eggs and a pinch of salt together in a small bowl
Heat 3 tablespoons of olive oil in a pan over medium heat
Fry the diced onions in the pan
Pour the egg mixture into the pan
As eggs begin to set, gently move spatula across the bottom to break the egg curds that begin to form in the pan
Cook until no visible liquid egg remains

MUSHROOM OMELET

Slice 2 medium sized mushrooms
Dice a small sized onion into small cubes
Whisk 3 eggs and a pinch of salt together in a small bowl
Heat 3 tablespoons of olive oil in a pan over medium heat
Fry the mushrooms and diced onions in the pan
Pour the egg mixture into the pan
As eggs begin to set, gently move spatula across the bottom to break the egg curds that begin to form in the pan
Cook until no visible liquid egg remains

VEGETABLE OMELET

Dice a small sized onion into small cubes
Whisk 3 eggs and a pinch of salt together in a small bowl
Heat 3 tablespoons of olive oil in a pan over medium heat
Fry onions and vegetables first; you can use any kind you like such as tomatoes, peppers or spinach
Pour the egg mixture into the pan
As eggs begin to set, gently move spatula across the bottom to break the egg curds that begin to form in the pan
Cook until no visible liquid egg remains

MUESLI

Make coconut milk
In a jar, pour 1 tablespoon of flaxseed oil, 4 heaping tablespoons of unsweetened shredded coconut and 2 cups of water
Use a blender and turn the ingredients into a milk-like liquid
Prepare the cereal
Mix 4 ounces of whole grain rolled oats, 1 heaping tablespoon of flaxseed, 1 tablespoon of raw almond, 1 tablespoon of walnuts and 1 teaspoon of raisins
Add some fruits
In a bowl combine the coconut milk, cereal mix and fruits
Use a small cup of mixed berries or dice a small unripe banana and a small pear

SIMPLE RICE RECIPE

Heat 2 tablespoons of olive oil in a pan over medium heat
Cook and stir rice in the hot oil quickly to toast the rice, for 2 to 3 minutes
Pour water over the rice mixture (twice the amount of rice) and bring to a boil
Reduce heat to low; cook until the water is almost absorbed, about 15-20 minutes
Cover the pan with a lid and turn the heat off
The rice will be ready in 10 minutes
Serving size is 3-4 ounces

HOMEMADE BREAD

Dissolve 2 tablespoons of salt in ½ cup of warm water
In a large bowl combine the ingredients:
 - dissolved salt
 - 2 pounds of coarse whole-wheat flour
 - 1 tablespoon of olive oil
 - 2 tablespoons of instant yeast
 - 2 cups of water

Stir until the mixture is thick and sticky. If it's not thick enough, add some flour. If the dough is too dry, add some water. Knead into a ball shape. Cover the bowl with a kitchen towel and let it rise for 3 hours.
Cut the dough into 6 equal pieces and shape each piece into a ball
Preheat the oven to 400 °F (200 °C)
Bake for one hour
Whole-wheat breads have a different texture than supermarket breads. They are very rich and dense; even a small piece will satisfy your hunger. Serving size is 3 ounces.

WHEAT SCONES

Dissolve 2 tablespoons of salt in ½ cup of warm water
In a large bowl combine the ingredients:
  - dissolved salt
  - 2 pounds of coarse whole-wheat flour
  - 13.5 oz of butter
  - 2 tablespoons of instant yeast
  - ½ cup of milk
  - 7.5 oz of sour cream (14% fat)
  - 1 large egg
Stir until the mixture is thick and sticky. If it's not thick enough, add some flour. If the dough is too dry, add some water. Knead into a ball shape. Cover the bowl with a kitchen towel and let it rise for 2 hours.
Make the dough ¾ inch thick by using a rolling pin
Use a 2-inch cookie cutter to form the scones
Preheat the oven to 400 °F (200 °C)
Bake for 45 to 60 minutes, depending on your oven
The scones are ready once the dough gets firm and the crust turns golden brown
Serving size is 3-4 ounces

HOMEMADE PIZZA

Dissolve 1 ½ teaspoons of salt in ½ cup of warm water
In a large bowl combine the ingredients:
  - dissolved salt

- 1 pound of coarse whole-wheat flour
- 1 tablespoon of instant yeast
- 5 tablespoons of olive oil
- 1 cup of water

Stir until the mixture is thick and sticky. If it's not thick enough, add some flour. If the dough is too dry, add some water. Knead into a ball shape. Cover the bowl with a kitchen towel and let it rise for an hour. Flatten dough ball to half an inch thick. Stretch out into a round and place it on a baking pan lined with baking sheet.

Prepare tomato sauce from crushed tomatoes. Always read labels. Make sure it has no higher sugar content than 4%. Don't use paste or ketchup. Add a teaspoon of oregano and crush 3 cloves of garlic into the sauce. Spread tomato sauce on the pizza dough and add the toppings of your choice. For example cheese, mushrooms, green peppers, artichokes, ground meat, sardines or eggs.

Preheat the oven to 400 °F (200 °C)

Bake for 30 minutes

Serving size is 10 ounces

Enjoy your pizza

GREEK SALAD

In a bowl, combine chopped romaine lettuce, green bell pepper, red bell pepper, tomatoes, cucumber, red onion, feta cheese and pitted black olives. Whisk together olive oil, oregano, lemon juice and black pepper. Pour dressing over salad.

CHICKPEA SALAD

In a bowl, combine diced green bell pepper, tomatoes, cucumber, avocado, sliced red onion, fresh parsley and canned chickpeas. Whisk together olive oil, vinegar, lemon juice, cumin, salt and black pepper. Pour dressing over salad.

SARDINES WITH TOMATO SALAD

Open a can of *sardines in spring water* and drain the liquids
Add two spoons of flaxseed oil

Place sliced tomatoes on a dish, season with salt, pepper and chives

GARLIC GREEN BEANS

Place green beans into a pan and cover with water; bring to a boil
Reduce heat to medium-low and simmer until beans start to soften,
about 5 minutes
Meanwhile in a separate pan heat olive oil over medium heat
Add crushed garlic, salt, pepper and chili flakes
Saute until garlic is fragrant, about a minute
Add the drained green beans and saute for 2-3 minutes until the beans
are coated with oil

FRIED MUSHROOMS

Peel mushrooms and remove stems
Crack and whisk an egg in a bowl
Pour flour and bread crumbs into two separate bowls
First coat the mushrooms in flour, then in egg, and lastly in bread
crumbs
Heat olive oil in a deep heavy bottom pan
Deep fry the mushrooms until they are golden brown
Dry mushrooms on a kitchen towel and sprinkle with salt

MIXED SALAD

Slice tomatoes, green pepper, cucumber and radish
Whisk together one part of flaxseed oil, four parts of vinegar, salt and
black pepper. Pour dressing over salad.

LENTIL SOUP

Place a pound of lentils in a bowl and cover with water
Soak for 15 minutes and drain water
Heat 9 tablespoons of olive oil in a large pot over medium heat
Add 5 cloves of minced garlic, 1 diced medium tomato, 2 diced
carrots and 1 diced parsley root
Cook for 5 minutes; stir occasionally

Add 1 tablespoon of salt, 1 tablespoon paprika powder and a pinch of
black pepper
Add lentils
Add 1.5 quarts (liters) of water
Cook until lentils are soft (approximately 30 minutes)

SPLIT PEA SOUP

Place a pound of dried split peas in a bowl and cover with water
Soak for 15 minutes and drain water
Heat 9 tablespoons of olive oil in a large pot over medium heat
Add 5 cloves of minced garlic, 1 diced medium onion, 1 diced
medium tomato, 1 diced carrot and half a teaspoon of cumin seeds
Cook for 5 minutes; stir occasionally
Add 1 tablespoon of salt, 1 tablespoon paprika powder, 1 bay leaf,
half a teaspoon of thyme and a pinch of black pepper
Add peas
Add 2 quarts (liters) of water
Cook until peas are soft (approximately 30 minutes)

GREEN PEA SOUP

Heat 9 tablespoons of olive oil in a large pot over medium heat
Add 1 diced medium onion, 3 diced carrots and 3 diced parsley roots
Cook for 8 minutes; stir occasionally
Add a tablespoon of flour
Cook for one more minute
Add 1.5 pounds of green peas
Add 1.5 quarts (liters) of water
Add 1 tablespoon of salt, 1 tablespoon of paprika powder and a pinch
of black pepper
Cook until peas are soft (approximately 30 minutes)
Cut a handful of parsley leaf into the soup

BEAN SOUP

Place a pound of dry beans in a bowl and cover with triple amount of
water

Soak overnight and drain water
Heat 9 tablespoons of olive oil in a large pot over medium heat
Add 5 cloves of minced garlic, 1 diced medium onion, 2 diced
carrots, 2 diced parsley roots, half a celery root, 1 diced green pepper,
1 diced tomato, 2 tablespoons of paprika powder, 1 tablespoon of salt
and a pinch of black pepper
Cook for 5 minutes; stir occasionally
Add beans
Add 2 quarts (liters) of water
Cook until beans are soft (approximately 45 minutes)

MUSHROOM SOUP

Heat 9 tablespoons of olive oil in a large pot over medium heat
Add 1 clove of minced garlic, 1 diced medium onion, 2 diced carrots,
2 diced parsley roots, 1 diced green pepper and 1 diced tomato
Cook for 5 minutes; stir occasionally
Add 2 pounds of mixed mushrooms
Add 2 tablespoons of paprika powder, 1 tablespoon of salt, a pinch of
marjoram, a pinch of thyme and black pepper
Add 1.5 quarts (liters) of water
Cook for 25 minutes
Add 2 tablespoons of sour cream and boil for 2 more minutes

PUMPKIN SOUP

Heat 5 tablespoons of olive oil in a large pot over medium heat
Add 5 cloves of minced garlic, 1 teaspoon of grated ginger, and ½
teaspoon of cumin seeds
Cook for 1 minute; stir continuously
Add 2 pounds of peeled and diced pumpkins
Add 1.5 quarts (liters) of water
Add 2 tablespoons of turmeric, 1 tablespoon of garam masala (Indian
spice mixture), 1 teaspoon of coriander powder and a pinch of black
pepper
Boil until pumpkin becomes tender (approximately 25 minutes)
Remove from heat and use a stick blender to blend until smooth

Add 6 ounces of table cream
Simmer for 2 more minutes

CHICKEN SOUP

Put the whole chicken, 5 carrots, 3 parsley roots, half a celery root, 2 medium onions, 2 cloves of garlic, 1 tomato, 1 green pepper, 2 tablespoons of salt and ½ tablespoon of whole black peppers in a large soup pot and cover with cold water. Cover with a lid, heat and simmer until the chicken meat falls off of the bones, between 1 and 2 hours. Take everything out of the pot. Strain the soup. Pick the meat off of the bones and chop the vegetables and serve them together with the broth.

FRIED CHICKEN BREAST

Cut chicken breast into half-inch slices and season with salt and pepper
Crack and whisk an egg in a bowl
Pour flour and bread crumbs into two separate bowls
First coat the chicken breasts in flour, then in egg, and lastly in bread crumbs
Heat olive oil in a deep heavy bottom pan
Deep fry the chicken breasts each side for 2-3 minutes until they are golden brown
Dry chicken breasts on a kitchen towel

GRILLED CHICKEN

Combine olive oil, dijon mustard, Worcestershire sauce, lemon juice, salt, paprika powder, black pepper and crushed garlic in a bowl
Add chicken slices and toss well to combine
Marinate for least 2 hours
Preheat grill to medium high heat
Place chicken on the grill for 3-4 minutes each side or until no pink color remains

INDIAN CHICKEN

Combine tandoori spice mix with yogurt and lemon juice in a bowl
Add chicken pieces and toss well to combine
Marinate for least 2 hours
Preheat oven to 385 °F (195 °C)
Line a pan with aluminum foil
Place marinated chicken pieces into the pan
Bake for 15 minutes and then coat the meat with the marinade by
using a spatula
Flip over the chicken and coat the other half with the rest of the
marinade and bake for another 15 minutes.

DEEP FRIED BREADED COD

Season the fish with salt and pepper
Crack and whisk an egg in a bowl
Pour flour and bread crumbs into two separate bowls
First coat the fish in flour, then in egg, and lastly in bread crumbs
Heat olive oil in a deep heavy bottom pan
Deep fry the fish each side for about 2 minutes until they are golden
brown
Dry fish on a kitchen towel

FRIED SALMON / TROUT / TILAPIA

Season the fish with salt, pepper, and lemon juice
Heat olive oil in a deep heavy bottom pan
Pan fry salmon for 4-5 minutes each side
Trout and tilapia requires 3-4 minutes depending on thickness

52

HOW I LOST 42 POUNDS IN 80 DAYS

THE AUTHOR'S STORY

I was a normal-weight kid until the last year of high school. Although I've never been an athletic type, once in a while, I participated in medium-intensity, sport activities that required a certain level of endurance, such as swimming or running longer distances. However, things started to change shortly after I turned 17, when I got my driver's license. I gradually developed a very bad, sedentary lifestyle. I stopped occasional exercising and would drive literally everywhere. Virtually, I did not walk at all except for those short distances between the door of my house and the door of my car. My family often teased me, "You would even drive to the washroom if it were possible". In addition to my unprecedented laziness, I adopted a second bad habit as well: I got addicted to sugar-sweetened beverages, especially Coca Cola. I used to drink Coke as normal people would drink bottled water: 1 to 2 liters every single day. My diet was based on massive amounts of refined carbohydrates: sugar from Coca Cola, white bread, pasta, white rice and potato. Although, before the end of high school, I did not notice any significant change and weighed pretty much the same. During the first year of university, the numbers on the scale began to creep upward. By the age of 19, I had gained 22 pounds. In my mid 20's, with an extra 58 pounds, I became heavier than ever in my life.

At that point, I finally acknowledged that I had become obese and had to do something about it. That was the beginning of my hopeless battle against obesity, which lasted for a quarter of a century. Although I didn't have any serious health conditions, I felt miserable. I had the worst possible type of obesity: most of my body fat was concentrated in the abdominal region. I grew a huge belly and looked like a 9-month-pregnant woman. I was always tired, couldn't walk longer distances without exhaustion, and lost the ability to run or swim. My weight problem bothered me so much that I decided to try a radical solution. I started a rigorous, calorie-restrictive diet. I quit Coke and cut back my food intake drastically. As a result of my self-torturing regimen, within a period of several months, I managed to lose 33 pounds. It was not easy; it took a lot of pain and suffering, but I finally did it. I was very proud of the results of my hard work. At the age of 25, this was one of the greatest achievements of my young life.

You've probably heard the saying "It ain't over until the fat lady sings". I was young and inexperienced; I did not factor in the "fat-lady-effect". I was very naive. I thought that I would remain lean forever, and simply went back to my old life. Although I strictly limited my Coca Cola consumption to no more than two glasses a day, I did not make any other significant changes to my lifestyle. Not surprisingly, within a period of a year or two, all the weight gradually came back, except for 4 pounds, due to the limited Coca Cola consumption.

I had to face the reality that man-torturing, calorie restrictive diets simply don't work in the long run. This time, I was looking for an easy solution. My family doctor prescribed *Xenical* tablets for me (other trade name is *Orlistat*). Those miracle pills helped me lose a few pounds, however after I quit taking the tablets, the weight shortly came back.

Until my mid 40s, I weighed pretty much the same. After two decades of obesity, I decided to start a strenuous exercise program. I did lap swimming, 2000-3000 meters every single day. I managed to lose over 10 pounds. After a short period of time however, it was clear to me that 60 to 90 minutes of intense training in the swimming pool every day is not the ideal weight-loss solution for an overweight middle-aged man. Once I cut back my training sessions to below 60 minutes a day, the weight I had lost just started coming back again. I simply gave up. I had to accept the fact that I was going to be obese for the rest of my life.

Back in those days, there were no such books like this one available. I had to rely on mainstream medicine's standard advice: *eat less, exercise more.* However, neither decreasing caloric intake, nor increasing caloric expenditure, worked in the long run. I have always been a person who likes to think outside the box. I love challenges too, so I set an ambitious goal for myself: to get back to my high school weight by my 48th birthday. This time, I wanted permanent results, no more upward creeping scale. I went through the scientific literature and laid down the foundations of a new weight-loss program.

I was the very first subject myself. My regimen was based on intermittent fasting and the complete elimination of refined carbohydrates such as sugar, white flour, and white rice. I also continued exercising: I did 30 minutes of lap swimming every day. Throughout the whole program, I managed to maintain a nearly linear weight loss of more than half a pound a day. By day 80, the weight I lost totaled 42 pounds. The protocol was so efficient that after completing the program, I just kept on losing weight even in the maintenance phase.

After 25 years of obesity, I finally managed to lose 55 pounds in total. Now I weigh the same as I did back in high school (this is not even my graduation weight, but that one that I weighed back in grade 10). My BMI went down from 31 to 21. I feel 25 years younger. I can run again. Climbing a hill is not a problem. The best thing is that not only have I lost 55 pounds, but I have also kept the same weight for years. If I did it, you can do it too.

53

IT'S YOUR TURN NOW

REGULAR DIETS ARE DESTINED TO FAIL

If you've come this far, you've probably already noticed that in the long run, conventional dieting simply does not work as expected. It doesn't matter what diet plan you follow or how hard you try: the weight you lose will still slowly come back within a few months or in a year. The whole concept of how mainstream science looks at obesity is wrong. Obesity is a very complex disorder. The most widely-accepted *calories in – calories out* model grossly oversimplifies the cause of obesity. In *The Formula for Weight Loss* chapter we saw that the question of *What causes obesity?* is much more complex than previously thought. Calories, nutrients, fasting, hormones, genetics, your lifestyle, and even the duration of your obesity have a significant impact on your body weight. Caloric intake is just one of the several *terms* of this very complex equation. By simply cutting back on your calories, you won't address the underlying cause of your obesity, and the pounds will sooner or later come back. Authors of regular weight-loss diets typically focus on reducing caloric intake only, but they often don't see the whole picture. That's why such methods simply fail in the long run. Instead of useless dieting, you need to do something else. You have to make radical changes in your lifestyle.

START A NEW LIFE

It doesn't matter how old you are, or how much you weigh now, it's never too late to start a new, healthier life. The inhabitants of *Sardinia, Icaria, Okinawa, Costa Rica* and the *Seventh Day Adventist*s in California are the healthiest and longest-living people in the world. These places have the highest number of 100-year-olds and many people grow old without diseases such as cancer, obesity, diabetes, dementia, or heart disease. Many of them remain fit and healthy until almost the very end of their lives. We can learn a lot from these people. Their healthy diet, moderate food consumption, simple lifestyle, physical activeness, the natural environment, and a purposeful life all contribute to their incredible health. Although we live in a fast-paced, modern world, and we cannot just go back in time and simply copy the lifestyle of the *Blue Zones* people, there are still a lot of new habits we can adopt in our own lives. The building blocks of a successful weight-loss plan have already been detailed previously. As a closing thought, let me summarize the three most important steps you need to take in order to achieve permanent weight loss and live an active, healthy life.

As the first step of building your own *health zone*, you need to completely eliminate junk food from your life. The meaning of junk food goes far beyond hot dogs, ice cream, and sugary soft drinks. You should avoid every kind of processed food, especially those ones with highly-refined carbohydrate content. Blacklist every single food item with added sugar, white flour, and white rice. *Chapters 22 to 39* will guide you through the jungle of the food industry and help you make wise choices on what foods are good for you and what you should avoid. If you make your own food, you will have full control over the single most important factor affecting your health. Even if food preparation may sound a little bit challenging for you, consider the health benefits of minimally-processed natural foods. You can find lots of practical advice in *chapters 46 and 49-51*.

The question *When to eat* is nearly as important as *What to eat*. With the proliferation of junk food products, snacking has become our regular habit. Instead of following the traditional eating pattern including breakfast, lunch and dinner, most of us eat 5 or 6 meals a day. The vast majority of healthcare professionals support the new habit of constant "grazing". We were given bad advice. Frequent eating is harmful rather than beneficial. Non-stop eating keeps your blood sugar and insulin levels continuously high. Elevated insulin levels lead to obesity. In order to achieve a permanent weight loss, you need to narrow down the eating window, the time period between the first and the last meal of the day. *Chapter 45* gives you a detailed guide on fasting and how to schedule your meals throughout the day.

Being involved in regular physical activities is the third cornerstone of your health. The world's healthiest and the longest living people in the *Blue Zones* are very physically active. However, they don't need to go to the gym in order to stay in good condition. They do long-lasting, low intensity, physical work instead, such as gardening and household chores that keep them busy all day long. Our physical inactivity is one of the major contributing factors to the 21st century's obesity epidemic. For those of you who have a sedentary lifestyle, being involved in regular physical exercise is indispensable to preserve your health and promote weight loss. You don't need to be an iron man or run marathons. Half an hour of medium-intensity workouts 5 or 6 times a week will significantly improve your overall health and assist in your weight loss. *Chapter 47* gives you some practical advice on exercising.

Whether you are a healthcare professional, patient, or an individual who wants to take control of their health, I hope this book has given you a new perspective on health and weight loss. It's your turn now. Don't let anything hold you back.

To remain updated visit the author's website:
www.thepermanentweightloss.com

Thank you for reading, and I wish you all a long, healthy life.

Thomas Torok, Ph.D.

ENDNOTES

1 http://www.who.int/news-room/fact-sheets/detail/obesity-and-overweight (accessed on June 12, 2018)

2 wsj.com/articles/SB10001424052748703580104575361281784399058 (accessed on June 13, 2018)

3 Hannah Ritchie and Max Roser (2018) - "Obesity". Published online at OurWorldInData.org

4 Shlomo Melmed. "Williams Textbook of Endocrinology". Elsevier. 2016

5 Hashem B. El-Serag and David Y. Graham. "Contemporary Diagnosis and Management of Upper Gastrointestinal Diseases". Handbooks in Health Care Co. 2009

6 www.arthritis.org (accessed on June 16, 2018)

7 Ashkan Afshin et al. "Health Effects of Overweight and Obesity in 195 Countries over 25 Years". The New England Journal of Medicine 377;1 July 6, 2017

8 https://ourworldindata.org/obesity#adult-obesity-by-region (accessed on June 18, 2018)

9 Amina Khambalia et al. "Prevalence and risk factors of diabetes and impaired fasting glucose in Nauru". BMC Public Health 2011, 11:719

10 Cynthia L. Ogden et al. "Prevalence of Obesity Among Adults:United States; 2011–2012". NCHS Data Brief No. 131 October 2013

11 Jennifer L. Harris et al. "Fast Food Facts: Evaluating Fast Food Nutrition and Marketing to Youth". Rudd Center for Food Policy and Obesity, 2010

12 "Health, United States, 2016: With Chartbook on Long-term Trends in Health". National Center for Health Statistics.

13 "How to Reduce Sugary Drink Consumption among Latino Kids". Salud America! Issue Brief, December 2016

14 Marian L. Fitzgibbon et al. "The Relationship Between Body Image Discrepancy and Body Mass Index Across Ethnic Groups" Obesity Research Vol. 8 No. 8 November 2000

15 James B. Kirby et al. "Race, Place, and Obesity: The Complex Relationships Among Community Racial/Ethnic Composition, Individual Race/Ethnicity, and Obesity in the United States". American Journal of Public Health, August 2012, Vol 102, No.8

16 Mark S. Tremblay et al. "Obesity, overweight and ethnicity". Health Reports, Vol. 16, No. 4, June 2005

17 Mary Gatineau, Shireen Mathrani. "Obesity and ethnicity". National Obesity Observatory. January 2011

18 Paul T. von Hippel and Ramzi W. Nahhas. "Extending the History of Child Obesity in the United States: The Fels Longitudinal Study, Birth Years 1930 to 1993". Obesity (Silver Spring). 2013 October

19 Gary D. Foster et al. "A School-Based Intervention for Diabetes Risk Reduction". The New England Journal of Medicine 2010;363:443-53.

20 Thomas N. Robinson. "Reducing Children's Television Viewing to Prevent Obesity". JAMA, October 27, 1999-Vol 282, No. 16

21 Cara B. Ebbeling et al. "A Randomized Trial of Sugar-Sweetened Beverages and Adolescent Body Weight". N Engl J Med. 2012 October 11

22 Juhee Kim et al. "Trends in Overweight from 1980 through 2001 among Preschool-Aged Children Enrolled in a Health Maintenance Organization". Obesity Vol. 14 No. 7 July 2006

23 www.nbcchicago.com

24 Kathleen C. Reidy et al. "Early Development of Dietary Patterns: Transitions in the Contribution of Food Groups to Total Energy-Feeding Infants and Toddlers Study, 2008". BMC Nutrition (2017) 3:5

25 Ryan W. Walker and Michael I. Goran. "Laboratory Determined Sugar Content and Composition of Commercial Infant Formulas, Baby Foods and Common Grocery Items Targeted to Children". Nutrients 2015, 7, 5850-5867

26 James A. Levine. "Poverty and Obesity in the U.S." Diabetes, Vol. 60, November 2011

27 https://en.wikipedia.org/wiki/Hunger_in_the_United_States (accessed on June 9, 2018)

28 Chicago Magazine. http://www.chicagomag.com (accessed on June 9, 2018)

29 Leslie O. Schulz, Lisa S. Chaudhari. "High-Risk Populations: The Pimas of Arizona and Mexico" . Curr Obes Rep. 2015 March 1; 4(1): 92–98

30 A. M. Kriska et al. "The association of physical activity with obesity, fat distribution and glucose intolerance in Pima Indians". Diabetologia (1993) 36:863-869

31 Jeanne M. Reid et al. "Nutrient intake of Pima Indian women: relationships to diabetes mellitus and gallbladder disease". The American Journal of Clinical Nutrition 24: October 1971, pp. 128 1-1289

32 Frank Russell. "The Pima Indians". Washington Government Printing Office, 1908

33 Amadeo M. Rea. "At the Desert's Green Edge. An Ethnobotany of the Gila River Pima". The University of Arizona Press. 1997

34 Timothy M. Frayling et al. "A Common Variant in the FTO Gene Is Associated with Body Mass Index and Predisposes to Childhood and Adult Obesity". Science. 2007 May 11

35 Lyla M. Hernandez and Dan G. Blazer. "Genes, Behavior, and the Social Environment: Moving Beyond the Nature/Nurture Debate". National Academies Press

36 Hermine H. M. Maes, Michael C. Neale, and Lindon J. Eaves. "Genetic and Environmental Factors in Relative Body Weight and Human Adiposity". Behavior Genetics, Vol. 27. No. 4, 1997

37 Albert J. Stunkard et al. "An Adoption Study of Human Obesity". The New England Journal of Medicine. January 23, 1986

38 Leslie O. Schulz et al. "Effects of Traditional and Western Environments on Prevalence of Type 2 Diabetes in Pima Indians in Mexico and the U.S." Diabetes Care, Volume 29, Number 8, August 2006

39 R. Passmore and Yola E . Swindells. "Observations on the respiratory quotients and weight gain of man after eating large quantities of carbohydrate" British Journal of Nutrition, 1963, 17, 331

40 Alfred W. Pennington. "Treatment of Obesity with Calorically Unrestricted Diets". The Journal of Clinical Nutrition. Volume 1, Number 5 1953

41 M. Hession et al. "Systematic Review of Randomized Controlled Trials Of Low-Carbohydrate vs. Low-Fat/Low-Calorie Diets in the Management of Obesity and Its Comorbidities". Obesity Reviews 10, 36–50 2008

42 Leah M. Kalm and Richard D. Semba. "They Starved So That Others Be Better Fed: Remembering Ancel Keys and the Minnesota Experiment". American Society for Nutritional Sciences, 2005

43 Barbara V. Howard et al. "Low-Fat Dietary Pattern and Weight Change Over 7 Years The Women's Health Initiative Dietary Modification Trial" JAMA, January 4, 2006—Vol 295, No. 1

44 Elham Moghaddam et al. "The Effects of Fat and Protein on Glycemic Responses in Nondiabetic Humans Vary with Waist Circumference, Fasting Plasma Insulin, and Dietary Fiber Intake". The Journal of Nutrition 136, 2006

45 W. C. Willett. "Dietary fat plays a major role in obesity: no". Obesity Reviews 3, 59–68. 2002.

46 Francesco P. Cappuccio et al. "Meta-Analysis of Short Sleep Duration and Obesity in Children and Adults". Sleep, Vol. 31, No. 5, 2008

47 Gilberto Paz-Filho et al. "Leptin treatment: Facts and expectations" Metabolism Clinical and Experimental 64 (2015)

48 Hiromasa Yamada et al. "Ghrelin Production, Action Mechanisms and Physiological Effects". Nova Science Publishers, Inc. 2012

49   Ahmed Saad et al. "Diurnal Pattern to Insulin Secretion and Insulin Action in Healthy Individuals". Diabetes, Vol. 61, November 2012

50   K. A. Varady. "Intermittent Versus Daily Calorie Restriction: Which Diet Regimen is More Effective for Weight Loss?" Obesity Reviews 2011,12

51   Carmen Piernas and Barry M. Popkin. "Snacking Increased among U.S. Adults between 1977 and 2006". The Journal of Nutrition . Dec. 2, 2009

52   Jason Fung. "The Diabetes Code. Prevent and Reverse Type 2 Diabetes Naturally". Greystone Books. 2018

53   KR Sonneville and SL Gortmaker. "Total Energy Intake, Adolescent Discretionary Behaviors and the Energy Gap". International Journal of Obesity (2008) 32, S19–S27

54   James F Sallis et al. "Education Program (SPARK) on Physical Activity and Fitness in Elementary School Students". American Journal of Public Health, August 1997, Vol. 87, No. 8

55   Erik O Diaz et al. "Metabolic Response to Experimental Overfeeding in Lean and Overweight Healthy Volunteers". Am J Clin Nutr 1992;56:641-55.

56   David S. Ludwig and Cara B. Ebbeling. "The Carbohydrate-Insulin Model of Obesity Beyond Calories In, Calories Out". JAMA Intern Med. July 2, 2018.

57   John W. Erdman. "Soy Protein and Cardiovascular Disease. A Statement for Healthcare Professionals From the Nutrition Committee of the AHA". Circulation. 2000; 102:2555-2559

58   John T. Flynn. "God's Gold. The Story of Rockefeller and His Times." 1932

59   Martha May Tevis. "Philanthropy at Its Best: The General Education Board's Contributions to Education, 1902–1964". Journal of Philosophy & History of Education vol. 64, no. 1, 2014, pp. 63–72

60   Big Bucks, Big Pharma: Marketing Disease and Pushing Drugs. Documentary Film, 2006 Producer & Editor: Ronit Ridberg

61   National Institute on Drug Abuse.   (accessed on July 27, 2018) www.drugabuse.gov/related-topics/trends-statistics/overdose-death-rates

62   NBC News.   (accessed on July 27, 2018) http://www.nbcnews.com/id/14944098/ns/nbc_nightly_news_with_brian_willi ams/t/cancer-docs-profit-chemotherapy-drugs/#.VYG0X_lVhHw

63   CBS News.   (accessed on July 27, 2018) https://www.cbsnews.com/news/probe-pharmaceuticals-in-drinking-water/

64   Richard Horton. "Offline: What is medicine's 5 sigma?" www.thelancet.com Vol 385 April 11, 2015

65   Ray Moynihan. "Who pays for the pizza? Redefining the relationships between doctors and drug companies. 1: Entanglement" BMJ Volume 326, 31 May 2003

66 Jessica J Liu et al. "Payments by US Pharmaceutical and Medical Device manufacturers to US Medical Journal Editors: Retrospective Observational Study". BMJ 2017; 359:j4619

67 Richard D Mattes et al. "Nutritively Sweetened Beverage Consumption and Body Weight; A Systematic Review and Meta-Analysis of Randomized Experiments". Obes Rev. 2011 May ; 12(5): 346–365.

68 Pett KD, Kahn J, Willett WC, Katz DL. "Ancel Keys and the Seven Countries Study: An Evidence-based Response to Revisionist Histories" http://www.truehealthinitiative.org

69 Ancel Keys et al. "Diet and Serum Cholesterol in Man: Lack of Effect of Dietary Cholesterol". The Journal of Nutrition. Received for publication November 3, 1955

70 Ancel Keys' letter to the editor. The New England Journal of Medicine. Aug 22, 1991

71 William B. Kannel, Tavia Gordon. "The Framingham Diet Study: Diet and the Regulation of Serum Cholesterol" The Framingham Study, Section 24

72 Katsuhiko Yano et al. "Dietary Intake and the Risk of Coronary Heart Disease in Japanese Men living in Hawaii". The American Journal of Clinical Nutrition 31 : July 1978

73 F. A. Kummerow et al. "The Influence of Egg Consumption on the Serum Cholesterol Level in Human Subjects". The American Journal of Clinical Nutrition 30: May 1977

74 Fred Kern. "Normal Plasma Cholesterol in an 88-year Old Man Who Eats 25 Eggs a Day". The New England Journal of Medicine March 28, 1991

75 William Osler. "The Principles and Practice of Medicine". 1921.

76 Cristin E. Kearns et al. "Sugar Industry Sponsorship of Germ-Free Rodent Studies Linking Sucrose to Hyperlipidemia and Cancer: an Historical Analysis of Internal Documents". PLOS Biology November 21, 2017

77 Yan Jiang et al. "A Sucrose-Enriched Diet Promotes Tumorigenesis in Mammary Gland in Part through the 12-Lipoxygenase Pathway". Cancer Res; 76(1) January 1, 2016

78 Maira Bes-Rastrollo et al. "Financial Conflicts of Interest and Reporting Bias Regarding the Association between Sugar-Sweetened Beverages and Weight Gain: A Systematic Review of Systematic Reviews". PLOS Medicine. December 2013 Volume 10 issue 12

79 Rasha Al-Lamee et al. "Percutaneous Coronary Intervention in Stable Angina (ORBITA): a Double-blind, Randomised Controlled Trial" The Lancet. November 2, 2017.

80 William E. Boden et al. "Optimal Medical Therapy with or without PCI for Stable Coronary Disease". The New England Journal of Medicine April 12, 2007

81 Kathleen Stergiopoulos et al. "Percutaneous Coronary Intervention Outcomes in Patients With Stable Obstructive Coronary Artery Disease and Myocardial Ischemia. A Collaborative Meta-analysis of Contemporary Randomized Clinical Trials". JAMA Intern Med. 2014;174(2):232-240

82 Nicole M. Avena et al. "Evidence for Sugar Addiction: Behavioral and Neurochemical Effects of Intermittent, Excessive Sugar Intake". Neurosci Biobehav Rev. 2008 ; 32(1): 20–39.

83 Jonathan Owen. "A Recent Study That Said Diet Coke Can Help You Lose Weight was Quietly Funded by Coca-Cola". The Independent. 17 Jan. 2016

84 Ameneh Madjd et al. "Effects on Weight Loss in Adults of Replacing Diet Beverages with Water During a Hypoenergetic Diet: a Randomized, 24-wk Clinical Trial". Am J Clin Nutr 2015;102:1305–12.

85 M. Yanina Pepino et al. "Sucralose Affects Glycemic and Hormonal Responses to an Oral Glucose Load". Diabetes Care, Volume 36, Sept. 2013

86 Center For Food Safety. (Accessed on August 19, 2018) https://www.centerforfoodsafety.org/issues/311/ge-foods/about-ge-foods

87 Sumio Kondo et al. "Intake of Kale Suppresses Postprandial Increases in Plasma Glucose: A Randomized, Double-Blind, Placebo-Controlled, Crossover Study". Biomedical Reports 553-558: 0-00, 2016

88 Mohd Faez Bachok et al. "Effectiveness of Traditional Malaysian Vegetables (ulam) in Modulating Blood Glucose Levels". Asia Pac J Clin Nutr 2014;23(3)

89 A Ri Byun et al. "Effects of a Dietary Supplement with Barley Sprout Extract on Blood Cholesterol Metabolism". Hindawi Publishing Corporation Evidence Based Complementary and Alternative Medicine Volume 2015, Article ID 473056,

90 whatsonmyfood.org/food.jsp?food=PO (accessed on August 23, 2018)

91 H. N. Englyst et al. "Classification and Measurement of Nutritionally Important Starch Fractions". European Journal of Clinical Nutrition. November 1992 46 (suppl. 2)

92 Diane F. Birt et al. "Resistant Starch: Promise for Improving Human Health". American Society for Nutrition. Adv. Nutr. 4: 587–601, 2013

93 Jiansong Bao et al. "Prediction of Postprandial Glycemia and Insulinemia in Lean, Young, Healthy Adults: Glycemic Load Compared with Carbohydrate Content Alone". Am J Clin Nutr 2011;93:984–96.

94 John C. LaRosa et al. "The Cholesterol Facts". Circulation Vol 81, No 5, May 1990

95 James D. Neaton et al. "A Case of Data Alteration in the Multiple Risk Factor Intervention Trial (MRFIT)". Controlled Clinical Trials 12:731-740 (1991)

96 Letter to the Editor. Further response from Hoenselaar.
    British Journal of Nutrition (2012), 108, 939–942

97 Dariush Mozaffarian et al. "Effects on Coronary Heart Disease of Increasing
    Polyunsaturated Fat in Place of Saturated Fat: A Systematic Review and Meta-
    Analysis of Randomized Controlled Trials".
    PLOS Medicine. March 2010 Volume 7 Issue 3

98 Ffion Lloyd-Williams et al. "Estimating the Cardiovascular Mortality Burden
    Attributable to the European Common Agricultural Policy on Dietary Satu-
    rated Fats". Bulletin of the World Health Organization 2008;86:535–541.

99 Ronald P. Mensink et al. "Effect of Dietary trans Fatty Acids on High-Density
    and Low-Density Lipoprotein Cholesterol Levels in Healthy Subjects". N Engl
    J Med August 16, 1990 323:439-445

100 C. Gómez Candela et al. "Importance of a Balanced Omega 6/omega 3 Ratio
    for the Maintenance of Health. Nutritional Recommendations".
    Nutr Hosp. 2011;26(2):323-329

101 A.K. de Freitas et al. "Nutritional Composition of the Meat of Hereford and
    Braford Steers Finished on Pastures or in a Feedlot in Southern Brazil".
    Meat Science 96 (2014) 353–360

102 Eric N Ponnampalam et al. "Effect of Feeding Systems on Omega-3 Fatty
    Acids, Conjugated Linoleic Acid and Trans Fatty Acids in Australian Beef
    Cuts: Potential Impact on Human Health".
    Asia Pac J Clin Nutr 2006;15 (1):21-29

103 N. Babio et al. "Association Between Red Meat Consumption and Metabolic
    Syndrome in a Mediterranean Population At High Cardiovascular Risk: Cross
    Sectional and 1-year Follow-up Assessment".
    Nutrition, Metabolism & Cardiovascular Diseases (2010) xx, 1-8

104 An Pan et al. "Red Meat Consumption and Mortality".
    Arch Intern Med/Vol 172 (No. 7), Apr 9, 2012 555

105 Yiqing Song et al. "A Prospective Study of Red Meat Consumption and Type
    2 Diabetes in Middle-Aged and Elderly Women"
    Diabetes Care, Volume 27, Number 9, September 2004

106 Joanna Kaluza et a. "Processed and Unprocessed Red Meat Consumption
    and Risk of Heart Failure Prospective Study of Men".
    Circ Heart Fail. 2014;7:552-557; originally published online June 12, 2014;

107 Martha W. Porter et al. "Effect of Dietary Egg on Serum Cholesterol and
    Triglyceride of Human Males". The American Journal of Clinical Nutrition
    30: April 1977

108 Diane Feskanich et al. "Milk, Dietary Calcium, and Bone Fractures in Women:
    A 12-Year Prospective Study".
    American Journal of Public Health June 1997, Vol. 87, No. 6

109   Constance B Hilliard. "High Osteoporosis Risk Among East Africans Linked to Lactase Persistence Genotype". BoneKEy Reports 5, Article number: 803 (2016)

110   G. Ursin et al. "Milk Consumption and Cancer Incidence: a Norwegian Prospective Study". Br. J. Cancer (1990), 61, 454-459

111   Janet W Rich-Edwards et al. "Milk Consumption and the Prepubertal Somatotropic Axis". Nutrition Journal 2007, 6:28

112   Andreas Daxenberger et al. "Increased Milk Levels of Insulin-Like Growth Factor 1 (IGF-1) for the Identification of Bovine Somatotropin (bST) Treated Cows". Analyst, 1998, 123, 2429–2435.

113   Sung-Woo Park et al. "A Milk Protein, Casein, as a Proliferation Promoting Factor in Prostate Cancer Cells". World J Mens Health 2014 August 32(2)

114   R.B. Elliott et al. "Type I (Insulin-Dependent) Diabetes Mellitus and Cow Milk: Casein Variant Consumption". Diabetologia (1999) 42: 292-296

115   Suvi M. Virtanen et al. "Cow's Milk Consumption, HLA-DQB1 Genotype, and Type 1 Diabetes". Diabetes, Vol. 49, June 2000

116   R. D. Briggs et al. "Myocardial Infarction in Patients Treated with Sippy and Other High-Milk Diets". Circulation, Volume XXI, April 1960

117   J. C. Annand. "Hypothesis: Heated Milk Protein and Thrombosis". J. Atheroscler. Res., 7 (1967) 797-801

118   Heinz Valtin. "Drink at least eight glasses of water a day. Really? Is there scientific evidence for 8 x 8?". Am J Physiol Regul Integr Comp Physiol 283: R993–R1004, 2002.

119   Philip R. N. Sutton. "Fluoridation. Errors and Omissions in Experimental Trials". Melbourne University Press, 1959

120   John A Yiamouyiannis. "Water Fluoridation and Tooth Decay: Results from the 1986- 1987 National Survey of U.S. Schoolchildren". Fluoride Volume 23, No. 2

121   Chun Z. Yang et al. "Most Plastic Products Release Estrogenic Chemicals: A Potential Health Problem that Can Be Solved". Environmental Health Perspectives Volume 119 number 7   July 2011

122   Neal D. Freedman et al. "Association of Coffee Drinking with Total and Cause-Specific Mortality". N Engl J Med 366;20   May 17, 2012

123   Xiuqin Shi et al. "Acute Caffeine Ingestion Reduces Insulin Sensitivity in Healthy Subjects: a Systematic Review and Meta-Analysis". Nutrition Journal (2016) 15:103

124 Nirmala Bhoo-Pathy et al. "Coffee and Tea Consumption and Risk of Pre-
     and Postmenopausal Breast Cancer in the European Prospective Investigation
     into Cancer and Nutrition (EPIC) Cohort Study".
     Breast Cancer Research (2015) 17:15

125 Arne Svilaas et al. "Intakes of Antioxidants in Coffee, Wine, and Vegetables
     Are Correlated with Plasma Carotenoids in Humans".
     American Society for Nutritional Sciences, 2004

126 S. van Dieren et al. "Coffee and Tea Consumption and Risk of Type 2
     Diabetes". Diabetologia (2009) 52:2561–2569

127 J. E. Enstrom. "Colorectal Cancer and Beer Drinking".
     Br. J. Cancer (1977) 35, 674

128 Stella G Muthuri et al. "Beer and Wine Consumption and Risk of Knee or
     Hip Osteoarthritis: a Case Control Study".
     Arthritis Research & Therapy (2015) 17:23

129 Jiansong Bao et al. "Prediction of Postprandial Glycemia and Insulinemia in
     Lean, Young, Healthy Adults: Glycemic Load Compared with Carbohydrate
     Content Alone". Am J Clin Nutr 2011;93:984–96

130 Andreas Gerloff et al. "Beer and its Non-Alcoholic Compounds: Role in
     Pancreatic Exocrine Secretion, Alcoholic Pancreatitis and Pancreatic
     Carcinoma". Int. J. Environ. Res. Public Health 2010, 7, 1093-1104

131 https://www.greenpeace.org/archive-international/en/press/releases/2007/
     anheuser-busch-using-experimen/   (accessed on September 19, 2018)

132 S. Milligan et al. "Oestrogenic Activity of the Hop Phyto-oestrogen,
     8-prenylnaringenin". Reproduction (2002) 123, 235–242

133 www.acs.org/content/acs/en/pressroom/newsreleases/2013/april/widely-
     used-filtering-material-adds-arsenic-to-beers.html (accessed on 9/19, 2018)

134 "Dietary Reference Intakes for Water, Potassium, Sodium, Chloride, and
     Sulfate". The National Academies Press. 2005. www.nap.edu.

135 Intersalt Cooperative Research Group. "Intersalt: an International Study of
     Electrolyte Excretion and Blood Pressure. Results for 24 Hour Urinary
     Sodium and Potassium Excretion". BMJ Volume 297 30 July 1988

136 Feng J He et al. "Effect of Longer Term Modest Salt Reduction on Blood
     Pressure: Cochrane Systematic Review and Meta-Analysis of Randomised
     Trials". BMJ 2013; 346 : f1325

137 Jay M. Sullivan et al. "Hemodynamic Effects of Dietary Sodium in Man.
     A Preliminary Report". Hypertension Vol 2, No 4, July-August 1980

138 Purnendu K. Dasgupta et al. "Iodine Nutrition: Iodine Content of Iodized Salt
     in the United States". Environ. Sci. Technol. 2008, 42, 1315–1323

139 Ancel Keys Austin F. Henschel. "Vitamin Supplementation of U. S. Army Rations in Relation to Fatigue and the Ability to do Muscular Work." The Journal of Nutrition, Volume 23, Issue 3, 1 March 1942, Pages 259–269

140 David J.A. Jenkins et al. "Supplemental Vitamins and Minerals for CVD Prevention and Treatment." Journal of the American College of Cardiology Vol. 71 , No. 2 2, 2 0 1 8

141 Marta Ebbing et al. "Cancer Incidence and Mortality After Treatment With Folic Acid and Vitamin B12". JAMA, November 18, 2009-Vol 302, No. 19

142 A. Catharine Ross, Christine L. Taylor, Ann L. Yaktine, Heather B. Del Valle. "Dietary Reference Intakes for Calcium and Vitamin D". The National Academies Press, 2011

143 Curtiss D Hunt, LuAnn K Johnson. "Calcium Requirements: New Estimations for Men and Women by Cross-sectional Statistical Analyses of Calcium Balance Data from Metabolic Studies." Am J Clin Nutr 2007;86:1054–63.

144 Rebecca D. Jackson et al. "Calcium plus Vitamin D Supplementation and the Risk of Fractures". N Engl J Med 2006;354:669-83.

145 Constance B Hilliard. "High Osteoporosis Risk Among East Africans Linked to Lactase Persistence Genotype." BoneKEy Reports 5, Article number: 803

146 Tomoo Kondo et al. "Vinegar Intake Reduces Body Weight, Body Fat Mass, and Serum Triglyceride Levels in Obese Japanese Subjects." Biosci. Biotechnol. Biochem., 73 (8), 1837–1843, 2009

147 National Center for Health Statistics. (Accessed on December 3, 2018) https://www.cdc.gov/nchs/fastats/leading-causes-of-death.htm

148 Selçuk Dağdelen, Tomris Erbaş. "Disease of the Sultans: Metabolic Syndrome in Ottoman Dynasty". Hacettepe University, Ankara , Turkey

149 Dan Buettner. "The Blue Zones Solution". National Geographic Society,2015

150 Caldwell B Esselstyn. "A Plant-Based Diet and Coronary Artery Disease: a Mandate for Effective Therapy". Journal of Geriatric Cardiology (2017) 14

151 Patrick L. Hill, Nicholas A. Turiano. "Purpose in Life as a Predictor of Mortality across Adulthood". Psychol Sci. 2014 July ; 25(7): 1482–1486

152 Menelaos L. Batrinos. "The length of life and eugeria in classical Greece" Hormones 2008, 7(1):82-83

153 P Burton, HJ Lightowler. "The Impact of Freezing and Toasting on the glycaemic Response of White Bread". European Journal of Clinical Nutrition (2008) 62, 594–599.

www.ingramcontent.com/pod-product-compliance
Lightning Source LLC
Chambersburg PA
CBHW030237030426
42336CB00009B/133